Birgitta Langhammer

Physiotherapy after Stroke - a Lifetime Endeavour

Birgitta Langhammer

Physiotherapy after Stroke - a Lifetime Endeavour

Why and How

VDM Verlag Dr. Müller

Imprint

Bibliographic information by the German National Library: The German National Library lists this publication at the German National Bibliography; detailed bibliographic information is available on the Internet at http://dnb.d-nb.de.

Cover image: www.purestockx.com

Publisher:
VDM Verlag Dr. Müller Aktiengesellschaft & Co. KG , Dudweiler Landstr. 125 a, 66123 Saarbrücken, Germany,
Phone +49 681 9100-698, Fax +49 681 9100-988,
Email: info@vdm-verlag.de

Zugl.: Oslo, University of Oslo,Faculty of Medicine, Diss., 2007

Produced in USA and UK by:
Lightning Source Inc., La Vergne, Tennessee, USA
Lightning Source UK Ltd., Milton Keynes, UK
BookSurge LLC, 5341 Dorchester Road, Suite 16, North Charleston, SC 29418, USA

ISBN: 978-3-639-07133-7

Acknowledgements 3
Original publications 5
List of abbreviations 6
1   Background 7
    1.1 Stroke - General aspects 7
    1.2   Acute stroke 8
        1.2.1   Recovery after stroke 9
        1.2.2. Predictors of recovery after stroke 10
    1.3   Chronic stroke 10
    1.4   Classification of functioning, disability and health 12
        1.3.1   Definitions of ICF components in the context of health 13
    1.5   Impairments, activity limitations and participation restrictions 14
        1.5.1   Impairments after stroke 14
        1.5.2   Activity limitations after stroke 17
        1.5.3   Participation restrictions after stroke 18
        1.5.4   Environmental factors – effects on outcome after stroke 18
        1.5.5   Personal factors – effects on outcome after stroke 19
    1.6   Physiotherapy – definition 19
        1.6.1   Conceptual framework for clinical practice 20
        1.6.2   Motor control 20
        1.6.3   Theories of motor control 20
        1.6.4   Physiotherapy in stroke rehabilitation 21
        1.6.5   Evidence-based physiotherapy in stroke rehabilitation 23
2   Aims 24
3   Subjects 25
    3.1   Inclusion and exclusion criteria 25
4   Design and methods 26
    4.1   Design 26
    4.2   Methods 27
        4.2.1   Outcome measures 27
        4.2.2. Test occasions in the different studies 30
        4.2.3   Statistical methods 31
        4.3.4   Ethical considerations 32
5   Results 32
    5.1   Study I 32
    5.2 Study II 33
    5.3 Study III 35
    5.4   Study IV 38
6   General discussion 42
    6.1   Design 42
    6.2   Methods 43
        6.2.1   Patient selection 43
        6.2.2   Outcome measures 44
        6.2.3   Statistical approach 47
    6.3   Discussion - Results 48
        6.3.1   Bobath or Motor Relearning Programme? (study I) 48
        6.3.2   Bobath or Motor Relearning Programme? A follow-up (study II) 50

6.3.3   The relation between gait velocity and static and dynamic balance in the early rehabilitation of patients with acute stroke (study III) 51

6.3.4   Stroke patients and long-term training: is it worthwhile? A randomised comparison of two different training strategies after rehabilitation (study IV) 52

7   Conclusions and clinical implications... 55

8   Suggestions for further research.. 56

9   Reference List 58

Attachments... 79

Acknowledgements

This thesis has been made possible through the inspiring support and shared knowledge of many people in different clinical and teaching settings. To all those who in any way have contributed to this work, I would like to express my sincere appreciation. I am particularly grateful to:

−   all patients and their relatives, without whose participation, interest and patience this study would not have been accomplished;

-    my colleagues and friends at the physiotherapy department at Asker and Bærum Hospital for moral and practical support through all these years;

-    all co-workers and colleagues in Asker and Bærum communities and private practices, whose help and positive support was crucial for the follow-up intervention;

-    the Faculty of Health, Oslo University College, for financial support.

My special thanks are due to the following persons:

Professor Birgitta Lindmark, my co-author and main scientific supervisor for generously sharing her scientific knowledge, for her advice, support, and quick replies to my questions, and for her great interest in my work. It has been an inspiration to work with you and I thank you for your creative criticism, enthusiasm and patience.

Professor Johan K Stanghelle, my co-author and scientific supervisor for generous support, great interest in my work and for believing in me from the beginning. Thank you for expertly guiding and accompanying me through this journey of academic experiences and for your confidence in my ability.

My colleagues Audhild Tørstad and Else Dreyer at the stroke unit, Asker and Bærum Hospital, for their valuable assistance and collaboration in the recruiting of patients to the stroke studies, and all other co-workers and colleagues at the same unit for their positive support.

Maud Marsden, for excellent linguistic revisions and proposals.

Dr Astrid Bergland, colleague and friend for her interest, valuable discussions, creative criticism and cheerful support throughout the years.

Study leader Nina Bugge-Rigault, The Faculty of Health Sciences, Physiotherapy programme, Oslo University College, for moral support through this process of academic endeavour.

And especially to my dear family:

My husband Erik for being there, for love, support and for bringing me to Norway!

My children: Anna Karolin, Bjørn, Magnus, Frode, Jarle and Ellen Bera, for joy, inspiration, love and pleasure. My best motivators and sweetest companions!
My dear mother and sister for being strong female models, always encouraging and supportive!

Original publications

This thesis is based on the following original papers, which will be referred to by their roman numbers:

I.   Langhammer B, Stanghelle JK. Bobath or Motor Relearning Programme? A comparison of two different approaches of physiotherapy in stroke rehabilitation: a randomized controlled study. Clinical Rehabilitation 2000; 14(4):361-369.

II.   Langhammer B, Stanghelle JK. Bobath or Motor Relearning Programme? A follow-up one and four years post stroke. Clinical Rehabilitation 2003; 17(7):731-734.

III. Langhammer B, Lindmark B, Stanghelle JK. The relation between gait velocity and static and dynamic balance in the early rehabilitation of patients with acute stroke. Advances in Physiotherapy 2006; 8 (2):60-65.

IV. Langhammer B, Stanghelle JK, Lindmark B. Stroke patients and long term training: is it worth while? Comparison of two different ways of training after rehabilitation. Accepted for publication in Clinical Rehabilitation.

List of abbreviations

ADL	Activities of Daily Living
BBS	Berg Balance Scale
BI	Barthel Index of Activities of Daily Living
BOS	Base Of Support
CNS	Central Nervous System
COG	Centre Of Gravity
COM	Centre Of Mass
CT	Computed Tomography
EBM	Evidence Based Medicine
EBP	Evidence Based Practice
EMG	Electromyography
HRQL	Health-Related Quality of Life
I-ADL	Instrumental Activities of Daily Living
ICF	International Classification of Functions
ICD	International Classification of Disease
IG	Intensive exercise group
MAS	Motor Assessment Scale
6MWT	6-Minute Walk Test
MRP	Motor Relearning Programme
NDT	Neuro-Developmental Treatment
OARS	The Duke Older Americans Resources and Service Procedures
P-ADL	Personal Activities of Daily Living
PNF	Proprioceptive Neuromuscular Facilitation
QoL	Quality of Life
RG	Regular Exercise Group
SD	Standard Deviation
SMES	Sødring Motor Evaluation Scale
TIA	Transitory Ischaemic Attacks
TUG	Timed Up-and-Go test
WCPT	World Confederation of Physical Therapists
WHO	World Health Organization

1   Background

1.1 Stroke - General aspects

Stroke is defined as "rapidly developed clinical signs of focal (or global) disturbance of cerebral function, lasting more than 24 hours or leading to death, with no apparent cause other than vascular", as defined by the World Health Organization (WHO) (1). Transitory ischaemic attacks (TIA) are brief attacks of cerebral dysfunction of vascular origin in which the symptoms disappear within 24 hours. Eighty-five per cent of all strokes are caused by thrombosis or embolus, 10 % are caused by haemorrhage and 5 % by subarachnoid haemorrhage (2).

The incidence rate of stroke in Norway is estimated to be 3.1 / 1000 (3). Approximately 13 000 -15 000 persons develop stroke per year and the estimated prevalence in Norway is 50 000 per total population, i.e. approximately 1% - 1.8% (4, 5). In comparison, the incidence of stroke in Western Europe is estimated to be < 100 / 100 000 for men and < 70 / 100 000 for women and in Eastern Europe and the former Soviet Union the estimates are 306-156 / 100 000 for men and 222-101 / 100 000 for women (6).

The introduction of computed tomography (CT) and better diagnostics of stroke are believed to have increased the reported incidence rates in the last decades (3). On the other hand, it is hypothesized that a more intensive treatment of hypertension has reduced these rates so that the incidence of stroke has been reported to be unchanged or only slightly increased over the last decades. Men are more likely to have a stroke than women, but this trend is reversed after the age of 85 years. In addition, the incidence increases with age and 70 % of all patients with stroke are over 70 years of age (3, 7).

Stroke is the third cause of death in Norway. However, there has been a reduction in deaths in the last decades, resulting in a higher prevalence (4, 8) (Fig. 1). That is, lethality has gone down in patients aged < 75 years, from 20 % in 1985 to 11 % in 1998, but remains stable among persons over 75 (9-10). This increase in prevalence will lead to an increased population living with stroke, in need of care and rehabilitation.

Figure 1: Differences in stroke mortality between men and women in Norway 1951 – 2003, all ages; 0 – 70+. Blue / dark line = men, pink / grey line = women

7

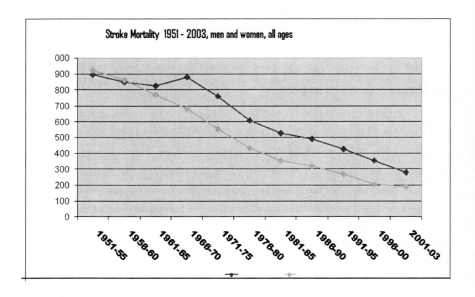

Stroke Mortality 1951 - 2003, men and women, all ages

1.2 Acute stroke

Stroke units have been established during the last decades, starting in the 1980s, with the aim of giving patients with stroke maximal care. Stroke units are defined as interdisciplinary stroke teams including specialist physicians, nurses, occupational therapists, physiotherapists, speech therapists and social workers in the acute hospital, organised as a ward or a mobile team in charge of patients with acute stroke (10). It is recognised that stroke units improve and hasten the rehabilitation of patients and it would be preferable that all patients with stroke could have access to this form of care (2, 11-14).

In the year 2005, 14 984 persons in Norway were registered with the diagnosis stroke according to the International Classification of Diseases -10 (ICD-10); G81 (0-9) (hemiplegia), I61 (1-2, 5-6, 8-9) (hæmorraghia cerebri), I62.9 (unspecified intracranial bleeding-non-traumatic, I63.0 (1-6, 8-9) (hemiplegia due to thrombosis, embolus) and I64 (apoplexia). Approximately 7600 of these stroke patients were treated in a stroke unit the same year (15). This means that in that year 51 % of all patients with stroke were admitted to the 48 existing stroke units in Norway (16). In comparison, Sweden has 80 stroke units and 73 % of all patients with stroke are treated in these units (9).

8

Stroke units in combination with the development of National Stroke Registers have led to improved stroke care. The National Stroke Registers target and register quality of treatment and lack of treatment of patients with stroke, contributing to easily accessible information and knowledge about stroke (11). A national register is currently under development in Norway with its centre in Trøndelag.(17).

National guidelines have been introduced in order to standardise and improve stroke care in several countries, e.g. Sweden, Australia, USA, Canada and England, to mention a few (18-20). The guidelines are based upon and developed according to evidence-based medicine, thereby providing recommendations for the best up-dated treatment and rehabilitation, which should warrant the quality of treatment for stroke patients. The national guidelines are the basis for clinical guidelines and these are developed locally to support clinicians in their daily practice. Clinical guidelines are defined as "systematically developed statements which help the practitioner and patient to make decisions about appropriate health care in specific circumstances" (21).

Impairments, activity limitations and participation restrictions in stroke patients will be discussed in more detail in section 1.5.

1.2.1 Recovery after stroke

Recovery after stroke is influenced by both intrinsic and extrinsic factors. A brain lesion affects both the anatomy and the physiology of the nervous system. The size of the brain lesion has the greatest impact on neurological recovery in both animal and clinical research studies (22- 23). All living organisms have an inherent capacity to self-organize throughout life and so recovery can be categorized as *spontaneous*, due to reparative processes, and due to *reorganization of neural mechanisms*, influenced by use and experience (24).

Spontaneous recovery probably represents the return to function of undamaged parts of the brain through resolution of local factors like oedema and the absorption of necrotic tissue debris and opening of collateral channels for circulation to the lesion area (25-26). This development is rather short in time, 3-4 weeks, and further recovery is explained by other mechanisms which underlie what is called *brain plasticity,* that is *reorganization of neural mechanisms.* Brain plasticity includes unmasking of pathways previously functionally inactive, sprouting of fibres from surviving nerve cells with formation of new synapses and redundancy in neural circuitry, i.e. multiple parallel pathways sub serving similar function

(27-29). This plasticity is thought to be driven by experiences, mobility, activity, interventions and the physical features of environment and its demands (24-32). Physiotherapy intervention can be said to be a driver of these plastic and dynamic changes with its focus on mobility and activities (33-35).

Patients who do not receive in-patients care could be seen as example of "spontaneous recovery". A study, which focused on patients with stroke that had not been admitted to hospital, concluded that; "Stroke patients not admitted to hospital have significant levels of disability which does not change substantially in the year after stroke" (36). The result of this study would indicate the importance of "drivers" of reorganization of neural mechanisms.

1.2.2. Predictors of recovery after stroke

Factors that have been identified as valid predictors of recovery after stroke are admission ADL score (37-41), urinary incontinence (37-38, 41-43), degree of motor paresis or paralysis (37-38, 43), age (37-41), loss of consciousness within the first 48 hours after stroke (37, 43), disorientation in time and place (37, 44-47), sitting balance (37-38, 41, 46), status following recurrent stroke (37, 40-41, 46, 48), level of perceived social support (37, 46-47) and metabolic rate of glucose outside the infarction area in hypertensive patients (37, 49). The methodological heterogeneity of many of these studies has been commented on by Jongbloed, who points out that; "It is important to identify factors that predict which patients have greater (or less) than predicted recovery. If interest lies with the prediction of function, at a particular point after the stroke, function should not be measured at discharge, since length of hospital stay varies enormously, but at a set time post stroke" (50).

Predictions can also be made regarding the pattern of brain activation (26). It has been shown that in patients with smaller injuries to the brain the ipsilateral hemisphere is activated to a greater extent (22). That is, a greater injury is associated with reduced laterality of brain activity (32, 51-52).

1.3 Chronic stroke

Approximately 70-80 % of all patients with stroke survive one year after the onset. The mortality rate thereafter is approximately 10 % every 6 months (53). Fifty per cent of the patients who survive a stroke display little or no reduction of function 28 days after the onset of symptoms, 20 % of the survivors have a major disability and 30 % a moderate disability in need of care, treatment and rehabilitation in the same period (54). Fifty per cent of the patients

10

with stroke report lower quality of life and 20-40 % depression and anxiety between 6 months and 7 years post-stroke (55-59). Secondary complications in chronic stroke

Secondary complications are not caused directly by the stroke but occur as a result of loss of function in one of the systems. Many patients with stroke experience secondary complications due to paresis / paralysis, reduced sensation, aphasia and apraxia (60-63).

In a study by Langhorne et al (60) approximately 85 % (n=311; 161 male, 150 female; mean age 76 years) of hospitalized patients with stroke experienced some form of secondary complication (Table 2).

Table 2. Langhorne et al. Medical complications after stroke: a multicenter study. Stroke 2000;31(6):1223-9.

Secondary complications	Patients with stroke (n=311) %
Recurrent stroke	9
Epileptic seizure	3
Infections:	
Urinary tract infection	24
Chest infection	22
Others:	
Mobility related falls	25
Falls with serious injury	5
Pressure sores	21
Thromboembolism:	
Deep venous thrombosis	2
Pulmonary embolism	1
Pain:	
Shoulder pain	9
Other pain	34
Psychological:	
Depression	16
anxiety	14
emotionalism	12
confusion	56

In other studies of secondary complications varying prevalence rates have been found. For example venous thrombus or embolism is reported in 20 -75 % of stroke patients (61-63), the occurrence of shoulder pain in 5-93 % (64-65) and / or the occurrence of general pain in 23-32 % (63-64, 66). In one study the prevalence of faecal incontinence in patients with stroke was found to be 11 % of after one year (67) and dysphagia has been identified during bedside evaluation in 40 % of patients with stroke (68). Depression is experienced by approximately 25-79 % patients with stroke (56- 58, 61), and in one study 19 % of the patients with stroke exhibited spasticity after three months (69). Although the prevalence is uncertain, there is agreement the type of secondary complications that might arise after stroke (61-69).

Inactivity as an indirect cause of stroke often leads to reduced endurance and strength (70- 75), which might be considered secondary complications. Reduced endurance and strength will in the long run directly affect the levels of activity and participation (76).

The differentiation between impairments directly related to stroke and secondary complications that arise as a result of such impairments can be diffuse. This in turn might lead to difficulty in discriminating between improvements of directly stroke-related impairments and reduction of secondary complications in chronic stroke patients. Some of the improvements in function that occur a long time after the stroke incident may well be explained by reduction of secondary complications, such as inactivity leading to reduced endurance, reduced strength, reduced balance and reduced mobility, to mention some (77).

1.4 Classification of functioning, disability and health

The World Health Organization (WHO) has developed the International Classification of Functioning, Disability and Health (ICF) to provide a unified and standard language and framework for the description of health. WHO has defined health as a state of complete physical, mental and social well-being and not merely the absence of disease or infirmity (World Health Organization, World Health Organization Constitution, Basic Documents. Geneva:WHO 1948) (78). The domains in ICF are health domains or health-related domains and are described in the perspective of the body, the individual and society in two lists: (1) body function and structures and (2) activities and participation (Fig. 2) (79).

Figure 2: The model of disability that is the basis of the International Classification of Functioning, Disability and Health (ICF)

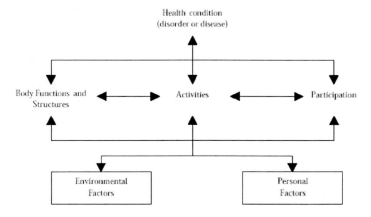

Functioning is an umbrella term encompassing all body functions, activities and participation. Similarly, disability serves as an umbrella term for impairments, activity limitations and participation restrictions. ICF also lists environmental factors that interact with all these constructs.

1.3.1 Definitions of ICF components in the context of health

Body functions are the physiological functions of the body (including psychological functions).

Body structures are the anatomical parts of the body, such as organs, limbs and their components.

Impairments are disorders of body function or structure such as a significant deviation or loss.

Activity is the execution of a task or action by an individual.

Activity limitations are difficulties in executing actions.

Participation is involvement in a life situation.

Participation restrictions are limitations in involvement in life situations.

Environmental factors make up the physical, social and attitudinal environments in which people live and conduct their lives.

Personal factors constitute the background of a particular individual's life and living, and comprise features of the individual that are not components of a health condition or a state of health, e.g. gender, age, overall behaviour pattern, coping ability and character style. Personal factors are not listed in the ICF.

1.5 Impairments, activity limitations and participation restrictions

Several body functions and structures may be impaired after stroke. These impairments may result in activity limitations and/or participation restrictions. Some common impairment is impaired motor function, sensory and perceptual deficits, impaired balance, cognitive limitations, aphasia and depression (39, 44-45, 48, 80-129).

1.5.1 Impairments after stroke

Motor function

Paralysis and/or weakness of one side of the body, i.e. hemiplegia or hemiparesis, are the most commonly reported impairment after stroke (80-82). Motor deficits in patients with first-time-ever stroke have been reported to be present in 77% in the upper limb and 72% in the lower limb (248). In the acute stage this weakness is caused by a disrupted neuro-muscular connection. In the chronic stages a secondary muscular weakness and atrophy in the functioning muscles may also be due to disuse (72-75, 80-82).

Tone - The upper motor neuron syndrome has been described as consisting of both negative and positive features (83-87). Negative features are decreased tone with signs of flaccidity-muscle weakness; slowness of muscle activation; and loss of dexterity. Positive features include increased tone which may lead to the development of spasticity (hyper-excitability) and resistance to passive movement (hyper tonicity). It has been recognised that increased muscle tone is due not only to increased reflex activity but also to intrinsic changes of the muscles (83), and thus Carr and Shepherd extended the description of *positive and negative features* by introducing the expression *adapted features* (84). Adapted features are a result of the positive and negative features, and are manifested clinically as muscle and connective tissue changes and altered motor patterns (24, 83). It is proposed that after three months a possible increase in resistance to passive stretch is mostly due to intrinsic changes of the muscle (83).

The prevalence rates of spasticity in patients with first-ever stroke 3 and 12 months post stroke have been reported to be as low as 19 % and as high as 38 % (69, 86). It has been suggested that spasticity may contribute to impairment of movement function and to limitation of activity, but it seems to have a less pronounced effect on health-related quality of life (HRQL) (87).

Incontinence - Urinary incontinence can affect 40-60 % of people admitted to hospital after a stroke, with 25 % still having problems on hospital discharge and about 15 % remaining incontinent at one year (88-90). Some reported prevalence rates of post-stroke faecal incontinence in stroke survivors are 30 % (7 to 10 days), 11 % (3 months), 11 % (1 year), and 15 % (3 years) (91).

Sensory function

Vision is an important modality for postural control and movement (92-95). Homonymous hemianopsia is a common symptom in stroke. In a retrospective study of patients with homonymous hemianopsia medical records were screened over the period 1989 to 2004. A total of 904 cases of this visual condition were found and of these, 629 (70 %) had a diagnosis of stroke. It was concluded that stroke was the most common cause of the syndrome (96).

Somatosensory impairment - is reported in up to 60 % of patients with stroke (97-99). Somatosensory modalities include light touch, vibration, temperature and proprioception. Reports suggest that somatosensory impairments are linked to poor spontaneous use of a limb, particularly the hand, which may lead to deterioration of the function related to hand movement (99-100).

Pain In a recent study in 297 patients with stroke, moderate to severe pain was reported by 96 (32 %) of these patients after 4 months. At 16 months, only 62 patients (21 %) had moderate to severe pain, but the pain intensity was more severe. The pain was persistent in 47 %, disturbed sleep in 58 %, and required rest for relief in 40 % of the patients (54, 66, 88). Pain after stroke is perhaps a neglected issue (101).

Shoulder pain occurrence among patients with stroke varies, with a reported frequency of 5 – 84 % (65, 102). Hemiparetic shoulder pain has been associated with weakness, immobility, abnormal muscle tone, glenohumeral subluxation and somatosensory impairments of the upper limb (65-66, 102).

Mental function

Impaired consciousness after stroke is a negative sign which is present in about 20 % of patients and is closely related to high mortality (44,104).

Emotional symptoms Thirty to 40 % experience depression and anxiety (46, 106-108).

Perceptual deficits are fairly common; 26-52 % exhibit neglect (45, 59) and apraxia has been observed in 28 % of all patients with a left hemisphere lesion staying in rehabilitation centres and 37 % in nursing homes (105).

Communication - impaired function of speech muscles may result in *dysarthria* which is reported to be present in 20-40 % of patients with acute stroke (109). *Aphasia* is defined as a disorder or loss of speech and language abilities caused by a brain injury. It is estimated that 20-38 % of patients with stroke suffer from aphasia in the acute stage, but this figure is reduced to 12-18 % six months after stroke (110-111).

Oral apraxia has been observed in 6 % of 618 patients with stroke, 9 % of those with a left and 4 % of those with a right hemisphere lesion (112).

Impaired balance – impaired postural control

Human balance is an operational construct, most often referring to the ability of a person not to fall. A mechanical definition of equilibrium is the state of an object when the resultant load (forces or movements) acting upon it is zero (Newton´s first law) (113). The position of the centre of mass (COM) or centre of gravity (COG) in relation to the base of support (BOS) is highly related to the static balance. In humans muscular activity is a mechanism used to counteract the forces of gravity and acceleration. This is known as postural control.

Postural control can be defined as the act of achieving, maintaining or restoring a state of balance during any posture or activity (93). In order to meet biomechanical challenges of tasks and environment, the postural control system needs adequate sensory input, efficient central processing and an effector system of afferent nerves, muscles and joints (114-115). Postural control strategies may be proactive, reactive, predictive, or a mixture of all three (93).

The main cause of balance disturbances after stroke is the lesion in the central nervous system (CNS), which affects information processing, integration of sensory input, and the effector pathways (93). Impairments with a negative impact on balance are disorders of the vestibular system (47, 93) and vision (94-96, 115), muscle weakness (93, 95), reduced muscle tone (93, 115), loss of range of motion (93) and impaired proprioception (93, 115). Prevalence rates of impaired balance after stroke have not been reported, but if balance is seen in conjunction with motor deficits, affecting postural control, a prevalence of approximately 70 % can be assumed in patients with stroke, but this is pure speculation (248).

1.5.2 Activity limitations after stroke

There is no internal hierarchical order of affect between impairments, activities and participation. Impairments after stroke may lead to activity limitations. On the other hand, patients with impairments may well be able to carry out activities and participate in all major areas in society and life. Independence in activities does not rule out the possibility of participation problems or problems due to environmental or personal factors (116).

Areas of activity where limitations might arise after stroke are defined by WHO/ICF as learning and applying knowledge, general tasks and demands, communication, mobility, domestic life and self-care (116-117).

Mental impairments and communication difficulties may influence learning/application of knowledge or general tasks/demands, or all of these, which might lead to both direct and indirect limitations of activities (118-119).

Mobility limitations such as transfer, gait and stair-walking difficulties can be major problems after a stroke (120-121). In a recent study by van Wijk et al, it was concluded that although many patients that survive a stroke achieve some form of independence in ambulation, few attain the same level of velocity and distance as their healthy counterparts of the same age (48). In the same study, however, it was found that the level of mobility attained during inpatient rehabilitation remained stable in the majority of patients with stroke over the second year after the onset (48). Only 12 % showed a decline in mobility, and depression was the only predictor of decline.

Dependence in activities of daily living (ADL) is reported to be highest immediately after a stroke, but is decreased one year post-stroke (39). It is generally agreed that the ADL improvements in most stroke patients are maximal within six months (122-123). However, there is a high risk of functional decline after the post-acute rehabilitation period (124-125). Functional decline in patients with stroke living in the community has been reported to be largely dependent on the clinical characteristics of the patient in question. Three of four analysed concomitant disabling conditions were associated with functional decline. These were pressure ulcer, urinary incontinence and hearing deficit, all of which can be prevented and possibly treated or modified, in contrast to the fourth condition, cognitive decline, which cannot.

17

1.5.3 Participation restrictions after stroke

It has been suggested that the participation domain may represent complex categories of "life behaviour" (126-127). The degree of participation is complex. Participation is conceived as a dynamic complex interaction between an individual's health condition, body functions, activities and external factors representing the circumstances in which the individual lives. It is related to quality of life (QoL) and is dependent upon environmental influences, as assessed in the community by self or proxy report, and the focus is on patients and caregivers. Participation involves the concept of autonomy, although the patient may not have to carry out the activities themselves. It also includes personal goals and social roles, and not only performance-based indicators such as upper and lower extremity function (128).

Restrictions in participation after stroke may refer to the degree to which the patient perceives that the disabilities after stroke restrict his or her ability to resume the pre-stroke roles that he/she had before the stroke (129). The restrictions vary, but they are connected with all levels of ICF (130). Jette et al. found three distinct concepts within the concept of physical functioning which they identified as conforming to the dimensions of Activity and Participation as proposed in the ICF. These distinct, interpretable factors which together accounted for 61.1 % of the variance in participation were labelled: Mobility Activities (24.4 %), Daily Activities (24.3 %), and Social/Participation (12.4 %) (126). Functional disability and mood disorders may independently contribute to restricted participation of patients post-stroke (129).

Only few studies have addressed participation restrictions in patients that survive a stroke, using the ICF framework. Studies dealing with the social impact of stroke have focused on QOL and have shown that restrictions in participation and depression are related to a reduced QOL, while social support can enhance QOL (131).

Studies of Instrumental Activities of Daily Living (I-ADL), which also reflect the participation level, have shown that stroke patients are to a great extent dependent upon relatives (132), that I-ADL are related to leisure activities (133), and that being male, unmarried, of high age, having severe motor impairment, having poor communication ability, and ADL dependency can be predictors of social inactivity 12 months post-stroke (129).

1.5.4 Environmental factors – effects on outcome after stroke

In animal research there is growing and convincing evidence confirming the role of an enriched environment in improvement of function (31, 134). This is very likely to be transferable to human beings and patients with stroke, in particular (135-137). In preliminary studies with the aim of leading to a definition of ICF Core Sets for stroke, 64 environmental factors were identified (116). Another study showed that ICF factor e399 (unspecified support and social network), under chapter e3, support and relationships, was the environmental factor of the ICF categories that was most used (117).

1.5.5 Personal factors – effects on outcome after stroke

Personal factors are not classified by the ICF because of social and cultural variations, which can make it difficult to interpret such factors with a global perspective. Personal factors, however, for example age, gender and hereditary characteristics, may have an impact on the stroke outcome. All these three are influential factors, but are impossible to alter or modify (37, 133).

1.6   Physiotherapy – definition

The 14th general meeting of the World Confederation for Physiotherapy (WCPT) adopted the following description of the profession. "The nature of physical therapy is providing services to people and populations to develop, to maintain and to restore maximum movement and functional ability throughout the lifespan. Physical therapy includes the provision of services in circumstances where movement and function are threatened by the process of aging or that of injury or disease. Full and functional movements are at the heart of what it means to be healthy ". Furthermore: "The nature of the physical therapy process is the service only provided by, or under the direction and supervision of a physical therapist and includes assessment, diagnosis, planning, intervention and evaluation" (Description of physical therapy adopted by the 14th general meeting of the World Confederation for Physical therapy (WCPT) May 1999, adapted final version at the extraordinary general meeting June 2003). The same general meeting decided that physical therapy and physiotherapy should be used as synonymous terms to identify the profession. Physiotherapy will be the preferred term used throughout this thesis.

1.6.1 Conceptual framework for clinical practice

Shumway-Cook and Wollacott introduced four key elements that they suggest will contribute to a comprehensive conceptual framework for clinical practice of physiotherapy (92). These elements are:

1) *The clinical decision-making process.* This includes gathering of information essential to the development a plan of care compatible with the problems and needs of the patient ; a plan consisting of assessments, analysis of assessments, development of short- and long-term goals, development of a treatment plan, implementation of the treatment plan and re-assessment of the patient and treatment outcome.

2) *Hypothesis-oriented clinical practice.* This involves systematic testing of assumptions about the nature and cause of motor control problems, and reflects the theories of a clinician regarding the cause and nature of function and dysfunction in patients with neurological disease.

3) *A model of disablement,* which imposes an order on the effects of disease and enables the clinician to develop a list of problems towards which treatment can be directed. An example of such a model is the WHO International Classification of Function, Disability and Health.

4) *A theory of motor control,* involving assumptions about the cause and nature of normal and abnormal movement, and include for example reflex-based neurofacilitation approaches or system-based task-oriented approaches.

1.6.2 Motor control

Rehabilitation practices reflect our basic ideas about the cause and nature of function and dysfunction (138 - 139). Motor control theory is part of the theoretical basis of clinical practice. A theory of motor control is defined as an idea of the nature and cause of movement (92). It deals with stabilization of the body in space, as this applies in postural and balance control, and with moving the body in space, as this applies to movement (92, 138 – 139). Motor control is usually studied in relation to specific actions or activities.

1.6.3 Theories of motor control

Different theories of motor control have been proposed throughout the years as researchers have added new knowledge to the understanding of the central nervous system, e.g. the reflex theory, the hierarchical theory, motor programming theories, the systems theory, the dynamic action theory, the parallel distributed processing theory, task-oriented theories and the ecological theory (92). A theory of motor control was presented by Shumway-Cook and Wollacott as a systems approach (140). This theory defines movement as an interaction between the individual, the task and the environment, where movement is the result of a dynamic interplay between perceptual, cognitive and action systems. Action systems are defined as the neuromuscular aspects and the physical/dynamic properties of the musculo-skeletal system itself (92).

1.6.4 Physiotherapy in stroke rehabilitation

Several studies have established that physiotherapy improves motor function and enhances mobility (141-144). Enhanced mobility contributes to recovery and it may therefore be assumed that physiotherapy after stroke is a promoter of recovery (36, 141-144).

Different physiotherapy approaches have been introduced over the years. Some methods are based on reflex and hierarchical theories of motor control such as the model of Rood (145), the proprioceptive neuromuscular facilitation (PNF) technique (146) and models developed by Brunnstrøm (147) and the Bobaths (148). Others, such as the systems approach (92) and the Motor Relearning Programme (MRP) (84), rely on recent theories of motor control and principles of neural plasticity (24, 84, 92, 149-156). Although all physiotherapy approaches improve motor function in one way or another, there is evidence to indicate that a systems approach is more favourable than reflex-hierarchical methodology in the acute treatment of stroke (143-144).

The improved function in the early stages of stroke is not self-supportive but will degenerate if not maintained (61, 124). Several studies have shown a reduction of motor and ADL function post-stroke when rehabilitation has been terminated (61,124-125).

Several studies indicate that what is practised is the function that is learned and improved; e.g. strength training with weights and aerobic exercise training improve strength and endurance, respectively, but do not automatically lead to an improvement in walking ability or more independence in ADL activities (157-166), or contribute to a higher degree of movement representations in the cortex (149 - 153).

Exercising "task activities" such as walking for example, on the other hand, can contribute to increased strength in leg muscles, increased endurance and increased representation in the cortex (76, 82, 161-164). However, these activities need to be exercised with a certain

21

intensity, variability and repeatability according to general training principles in order to give measurable results (149-156, 165-166). This supports the overall impression that a system-based approach coupled with application of training principles is favourable both in the acute and long-term rehabilitation of stroke (124,144).

It has been recommended the "global" approaches, a term introduced by Pollock et al, be abandoned because of the problems in describing, defining and consistently applying a complex range of interventions (167). It is probably sound and idealistic advice to concentrate on investigating clearly defined and described techniques regardless of their historical and philosophical origin (167). On the other hand, it must be kept in mind that current neurophysiological research and hypotheses will always be a basis for evaluating physiotherapy methods and techniques, and these theories can also be regarded as global approaches.

The global approaches in themselves are not problematic; the MRP, Bobath, PNF and Brunnstrøm techniques are all successful physiotherapy approaches (84, 146-148). All four methods are clearly documented and presented by their respective creators in books, with references to neurophysiological research that was relevant and up-dated at the time when the approaches were presented. These physiotherapy approaches may be compared to a brand in the marketing business. A certain value / definition is allocated to the brand / global approach and this, if successfully presented, will automatically be identified by all the potential users / therapists. The values and the key concepts of the four approaches mentioned are identified by therapists through the language, methods and philosophies used by the different physiotherapy approaches / "brands".

The problem arises when an attempt is made to change any of these approaches into something new, not realising the strength of the branding the approaches have. Inevitably "old" definitions and documentation cling to the name and for therapists this will create unnecessary confusion. A possible example is a method based on a reflex or hierarchical approach such as that of Bobath, where the therapists keep the basic philosophy and build their treatment on the old values; normal movement, key components, part training and just alter the references to the new neurophysiological research, for example the systems approach, in order to adjust and up-date the method to a changing world. The process may be justified by claiming that this is just a development of a therapeutic approach. In clinical practice this will create unnecessary confusion, as the two approaches have different philosophies, ways and strategies to deal with different clinical problems. Inevitably the physiotherapist will come to a point where he / she has to choose in accordance with her clinical belief and this is where "branding" and, hopefully, evidence-based practise will have a strong input.

At present, the most frequently applied "global approach" is the systems approach, defined as an interaction between the individual, the task and the environment, where movements are the results of a dynamic interplay between perceptual, cognitive and action systems. In recent years this has been the theory upon which most clinicians have based their understanding of the cause and nature of function and dysfunction in patients with neurological disease (92, 138-139). This is directly related to *hypothesis-oriented clinical practice*, as presented by Shumway-Cook and Wollacott (92).

A physiotherapist would ideally make use of hypothesis-oriented clinical practice, a model of disablement and a theory of motor control to form the basis of his or her clinical decision-making process in the practice of stroke rehabilitation. The actions in clinical practice and the choices of therapies will uncover any discrepancies between hypotheses, models of disablement, theories of motor control and clinical decision making (92, 138-139). That is: what the therapists say and intend to do and what they actually practise should ideally be compatible. The model of disablement and theory of motor control should serve as a control, so that the therapist can detect where the discrepancies may lie if the actions in practise do not harmonize with the model (92, 138-139).

1.6.5 Evidence-based physiotherapy in stroke rehabilitation

In recent years evidence-based medicine (EBM) (168) and evidence-based practice have been introduced into practical clinical physiotherapy. Evidence-based practice (EBP) includes the five components assess, ask, acquire, appraise and apply (169). EBP is dependent upon good research on clinical questions for development of clinical guidelines so that the practice at all times is of high standard and up-dated as a consequence of research. "Golden standards" of clinical research are randomised controlled trials, systematic reviews and meta-analyses.

The Cochrane Database of Systematic Reviews is an example of EBM and EBP, and some physiotherapy techniques in stroke rehabilitation are summarised in Cochrane reviews, e.g. treadmill training with or without body weight support (170), promotion of the recovery of postural control and/or lower limb function (167), acupuncture as a treatment of patients with stroke (171), amphetamine treatment on recovery from stroke (172), cognitive rehabilitation for spatial neglect (173), cognitive rehabilitation for memory problems after stroke (174), clinical use of electro-stimulation for neuromuscular re-training (175), and therapy-based rehabilitation services targeted towards patients with stroke living at home (176-177). The general conclusions drawn in many of these reviews are that there is a need for high quality randomised trials and systematic reviews to determine the efficacy of clearly described individual techniques and treatments in stroke rehabilitation.

There have been some good quality randomised controlled trials, however, in recent years (157, 144, 159, 178) that have made it possible to make some changes in clinical practice and that have led to national guidelines, which in turn may be revised when new research increases our understanding of the rehabilitation process in stroke patients (18-20).

In conclusion, it is generally acknowledged that physiotherapy enhances stroke recovery and that, as mentioned before, a systems approach, defined as an interaction between the individual, the task and the environment, where movement is the result of a dynamic interplay between perceptual, cognitive and action systems, is most beneficial (92, 143-144,154). There is consensus that treatment should start as early as possible, preferably in stroke units with a multidisciplinary team (11-13). However, there is no consensus on who will benefit most from rehabilitation, how intense and how long this rehabilitation should preferably be and how this therapy should be implemented. Furthermore, there is a need to be concise in the description of physiotherapy as applied in stroke rehabilitation, in order to evaluate different treatments and to reduce any discrepancies between what is said and what is being done (179).

2   Aims

The overall aim of this research was to evaluate the effect of physiotherapy in the acute and chronic stages of stroke in a model of disablement (ICF) and in the light of theories of motor control, and also to assess the influence of dynamic and static balance on gait in the early rehabilitation of patients with stroke. A further aim was to investigate the association between the patient's perception of his/her health-related quality of life and actual motor and ADL performance.

The specific aims were:

- to compare the effects of two physiotherapy approaches, the Motor Relearning Programme and the Bobath concept, in the acute and sub-acute stages of stroke and to evaluate the long-term effects of these therapies (studies I and II; papers I and II);
- to investigate the association between gait velocity and static and dynamic balance measured by Motor Assessment Scale items 3 (sitting balance) and 5 (walking), Berg Balance Scale (BBS) items 6 (standing blindfolded) and 8 (reaching forward) and the total score of Timed-Up-and-Go test on admission and at discharge from the stroke unit (Paper III);
- to investigate the effect of compulsory intensive physiotherapy training during four periods compared to treatment when required during the first year after first-time-ever stroke related to maintenance of motor function, grip strength, and P- ADL (Paper IV).

3   Subjects

All patients were recruited from the stroke unit at the local hospital. The patients were all admitted to the primary hospital for a geographical area covering a population of 155 000. About 260 patients were treated in the stroke unit per year. The mean length of stay in this unit is 7.9 days. In the year 2005, on discharge from the stroke unit 32 % of the patients were sent directly home, 19 % were transferred to nursing homes and 46 % were referred to the rehabilitation unit in the hospital or in the community; 3 % of the patients died before discharge.

The research described in this thesis is based on four studies carried out on three different study populations:

- Study population 1 comprised 61 patients with first-ever stroke, 36 men and 25 women, mean age 78 years (49 – 95 years) (studies I and II; papers I and II)
- Study population 2 comprised 57 patients with first-ever stroke, 31 men and 26 women, mean age 74 years (38 – 98 years) (study III; paper III)
- Study population 3 comprised 75 patients with first-ever stroke, 43 men and 32 women, mean age 73 years (38 – 98 years) (study IV; paper IV).

3.1   Inclusion and exclusion criteria

Inclusion criteria were first-time-ever stroke with neurological signs, computed tomography-confirmed stroke, and voluntary participation. Exclusion criteria were more than one stroke incident, subarachnoid haemorrhage, tumour, brain stem or cerebellar stroke and other severe medical conditions in combination with stroke. Patients fulfilling the inclusion criteria were consecutively included in the different trials as they were admitted to the hospital.

4   Design and methods

4.1   Design

Studies I, II, and IV were longitudinal randomised controlled stratified trials. Patients were randomised to one of two different groups by a person not involved with the patients or the treatment in the ward. Randomisation was performed with a dice; uneven numbers to group 1 and even numbers to group 2. Group 1 was the Motor Relearning Programme group in studies I and II and the intensive exercise group (IG) in study IV. Group 2 was the Bobath group in studies I and II and the regular exercise group (RG) in study IV.

Stratification was done according to gender and hemisphere lesion: the first male patient with a right hemisphere lesion and with an uneven number was allocated to Group 1, and the next male patient with a right hemisphere lesion was allocated to Group 2. The procedure with the dice was then used when the third male patient with a right hemisphere lesion entered the stroke unit.

In studies I and II, randomisation was performed as soon as the diagnosis was confirmed, after three days. The study was double-blind up to the three-month follow-up, when the seal was broken. The one-year follow-up test was not blinded.

In study IV, randomisation was effectuated at discharge from the acute hospital. The protocol was sealed for 1.5 years, from the start of the study until the last patient included was tested at the one-year follow-up. The study consisted of a double-blind-intention-to-treat trial. Neither the investigator nor the patients knew to which group they were allocated.

Study III was an exploratory study of walking capacity and static and dynamic balance in patients with acute stroke admitted to a stroke unit. The same inclusion and exclusion criteria as in the other studies were applied, but there was no randomisation. Sixty-one patients with acute first-ever stroke were enrolled consecutively in this study, with four drop-outs, leaving 57 participants in the study.

4.2 Methods

Performance-based and self-reported outcome measures were used. The measures were chosen to represent different levels of the ICF disablement model (180).

4.2.1 Outcome measures

The outcome measures were chosen to reflect the disablement process on the different levels of the ICF classification model, introduced by WHO (79). The outcome measures should also reflect the motor control theories influencing clinical practice in physiotherapy. The most dominant motor control theories in physiotherapy practice during this period have been identified as the reflex-hierarchical and the systems approaches (92,139). These two motor control theories were chosen as bases for different forms of treatment.

Table 1: Outcome measures used in the different studies.

Outcome measures	I	II	III	IV
Motor Assessment Scale (181)	x	x	x	x
Sødring Motor Evaluation Scale (182)	x	x		
Barthel ADL index (183)	x	x	x	x
Nottingham Health Profile (184) (health-related quality of life)	x	x		(x)*
Berg Balance Scale (185)		x	x	(x)*
6- Minute Walk Test (186)			x	(x)*
Timed Up and Go (187) (mobility and balance)			x	(x)*
Grip strength paretic and non-paretic hand (188)				x

* not presented here

In addition the following variables were recorded:

Study I: Length of stay, use of assistive devices, destination after discharge.

Study II: Use of assistive devices, patient's accommodation, use of services from the community, occurrence of new strokes, and other diseases.

Study III: No extra recordings.

Study IV: Patient's accommodation, help from the community and/or relatives, time from admission to discharge and civil status were recorded. Patients and relatives were also encouraged to keep track of the occurrence of falls and pain. The participants of both groups were interviewed concerning their training habits, their motivation to exercise, and whether and how they were doing exercises. Compliance to training programmes was recorded by the physiotherapist in charge of training and reported at the end of the study, after 1.5 years.

4.2.1.1 Tests

The Motor Assessment Scale is a test of motor function developed by Carr and Shepherd for assessment of individuals with stroke, using relevant and functional motor activities. It was designed for use in clinical practice and research (181). Eight functional activities are evaluated: turning in bed, sitting up, balance in sitting, standing up, walking, and activities of the upper arm, wrist and hand of the paretic arm. Each item is scored from 0 to 6. Hence the total scores range between 0 and 48. The test has been shown to have high inter- ($r = 0.89$ to 0.99) and intra-reliability ($r = 0.87 - 0.98$) and high construct-cross-sectional validity ($r = 0.88$ and $r = 0.96$) (189).

The Sødring Motor Evaluation Scale (SMES) is a test of motor function after stroke developed by Sødring. The unassisted performance of the patient is assessed and the scoring reflects a combination of quantity and quality of the movements (182). The instrument has 32 items, distributed among three subscales measuring leg function (SMES 1), arm function (SMES 2) and functions concerning trunk, balance and gait (SMES 3). Each item is scored from $0 - 5$. Hence the total scores range from 0 to 20 (SMES 1), from 0 to 70 (SMES 2) and from 0 to 60 (SMES 3). The test is valid and reliable (182, 190-191), with a high predictive validity in predicting residence at home or in an institution, and the results are obtained with the Barthel Index and and the Frenchay Activities Index one year post-stroke (191).

The Barthel Index of Activities of Daily Living (BI) is a test of primary activities for daily living developed by Mahoney and Barthel (183) for the purpose of measuring functional independence in personal care and mobility. The index includes ten activities of daily life: feeding, transferring from wheelchair to bed and back, personal hygiene, getting on and off toilet, bathing, walking on a level surface/propelling wheelchair, ascending and descending stairs, dressing, controlling bowels and controlling bladder. The items are weighted differently. The scores reflect the amount of time and assistance required by a client. A score of 0 (complete dependence), 5, 10 or 15 is assigned to each level, for a total score of 100. The test has high scores for inter- (r = 0.70 to 0.88), and intra-reliability (r = 0.84 and r = 0.98) and construct-cross-sectional validity (r = 0.73 to 0.77) (192-193). The BI scores in study IV were also dichotomised into lower (0 – 59) and higher scores (60 - 100). This estimation was based on the clinical guideline of a cut-off point of 60, which indicates a need for institutional care (194).

The Six-Minute Walk Test (6MWT) measures walking capacity and walked distance (m) and allows calculation of gait velocity (m/s) (195-197). The 6MWT is also used to assess exercise tolerance (196-196), thus measuring the functional exercise capacity (196). Gait velocity calculation has been tested for validity and reliability among healthy elderly individuals and patients with heart failure with satisfactory results (197-199). The 6MWT has also been used in studies including patients with stroke (200).)

The Berg Balance Scale (BBS) is a balance test developed by Berg et al, and consists of 14 items, scored from 0 to 4 (185). The total scores ranges from 0 to 56. It has been used in many studies and when tested has shown satisfactory reliability and validity (185, 199, 201-202). BBS is especially sensitive for detection of risks of falls in frail elderly persons. An overall score of less than 45 points, out of a maximum of 56, is associated with a 2.7 times increase in the risk of a future fall (92).

The Timed Up and Go test (TUG) is a functional mobility test used in the clinic to evaluate dynamic balance, gait and transfers. The test was further developed by Podsiadlo from the original Get-Up and Go test presented by Mathias et al (187, 203). The patient is asked to get up from a chair (46 cm high), with support for the arms, walk three meters, turn, go back and sit down. The physiotherapist monitors the time from the start to the end, when the patient is seated. The test is valid and reliable and has been used in several studies (193, 199, 204-205).

Grip strength was measured with a *Martin vigorimeter*, consisting of a manometer with rubber tubing and three different sized rubber balls: male, female / young and child size. The manometer gives the respective reading in bar = 1.019 kp/cm² (kp - kilopond). When taking the test, the patient has to squeeze the vigorimeter three times with all possible strength without seeing the gauge. The average of the three squeezes is then used. Normal values of healthy people are for male adult 0.8 to 1.3 kp (bar), and for female adult 0.7 to 1.2 kp (bar) (188, 206-208). Validity has been compared between the Jamar dynamometer and Martin vigorimeter and Pearson´s product-moment correlation was r = 0.89 for the right hand and 0.90 for the left hand (188). Test-retest reliability showed an intra-class correlation coefficient of 0.96 for the mean of three measurements on the dominant hand and of 0.98 on the other (208).

The Nottingham Health Profile (NHP) was designed with the aim of obtaining a subjective measure of health encompassing the social and personal effects of illness (184). The NHP consists of two parts. The first part consists of 38 questions relating to emotional, sleep, energy, pain, physical and social function with strictly yes or no answers. Each item carries with it a weight, based on the perceived severity of the item. Weight assigned to items in each dimension adds to a total of 100. A positive answer is associated with a particular weight, while a negative answer receives no score. Higher scores correspond to a poorer perceived health status. The second part consists of 7 yes/no questions relating to work, maintenance of the home, social life, domestic life, sexuality, hobbies and vacation. There are no weights for the second part of NHP. This instrument has been used in numerous studies (209-212). It has been tested for reliability (213-214) and validity (215) and has been found to be both reliable and valid in studies relating to stroke (212).

Compliance to the training programmes was recorded by the physiotherapists in charge of the follow-up treatment in study IV. Compliance was considered high in the intensive exercise group if the patients took part in all four exercise periods in the year post-stroke at least twice a week. Follow–up physiotherapy after the acute rehabilitation was minimal in study II (124), and therefore in IV any treatment after the acute rehabilitation in the regular exercise group was considered high compliance, since the expectations of such post-stroke treatment were low, in fact we expected as little such treatment as in study II (124). Information on the extent of participation in physiotherapy treatment of the two groups was also obtained through informal interviews on each test occasion concerning the patient's own training habits, their motivation for exercise, and whether and how they were doing exercises. Motivation was considered high if the participants did the exercises regularly, if they complied with the tests at different times during the year post-stroke and if they expressed a positive verbal opinion of the importance of exercise. This information was noted during interviews on the different test occasions and was compared with the actual training information from the physiotherapists, when the seal of blinding was broken at the end of the study.

Protocols for training were developed for study I (attachments 1, 2, 3) and for study IV (attachment 4).

4.2.2. Test occasions in the different studies

In study I the patients were assessed on the third day after admission to the stroke unit, and also after two weeks and at three months.

In study II the patients were assessed at three months, one year and four years post-stroke.

In study III the patients were assessed within three days after admission to the hospital and one day before discharge.

In study IV the patients were tested on admission, at discharge, and at three, six and 12 months post-stroke.

The tests were carried out by an experienced investigator, blinded to group allocation. They were performed in the general hospital, in the patients' homes and in the community service centres.

4.2.3 Statistical methods

The results of all studies were analysed in an SPSS programme, but different versions: 10, 12 and 13. In all analyses $p<0.05$ was considered statistically significant.

Study I: Means, medians and standard deviations (SD) were calculated for sum scores of MAS, SMES and BI, and means and SD for NHP. To evaluate group differences, Student's t- test was used. Group differences between test 1 and test 2 were also evaluated by analysing differences between two tests. Analysis of variance (ANOVA) for repeated measurements, with a Bonferroni correction, was used to assess differences in changes in motor and ADL function from test 1 to test 3 between groups. Differences between groups regarding gender, length of stay in the hospital, destination after discharge, use of assistive devices and the results of NHP, were tested using the Mann-Whitney nonparametric test.

Study II: Means, medians and SD were calculated for sum scores of MAS, SMES and BI, and means and SD for NHP. Student´s t-test for evaluation of group differences was used for MAS, SMES and BI. The results of NHP were tested with the Mann-Whitney nonparametric test.

Study III: Descriptive statistics were calculated for each clinical test. The paired t-test was used for gait velocity and TUG, and the Wilcoxon signed ranks test for related samples, for MAS and BBS items, and for comparing values on admission and at discharge. Spearman's rank correlation coefficients were calculated to check for associations between 6MWT and other tests. A standard multiple regression analysis was performed, where variables associated with 6MWT were entered into the model and run separately for each test occasion - test 1 and test 2. Preliminary graphical analysis was carried out to determine that all applicable variables met the assumption of normality and that no outliers existed. Thereafter a stepwise procedure was performed for each time moment, and a reduced model was analysed to test for an association between gait velocity in the 6 MWT and the independent variables BBS items 6 (standing blindfolded) and 8 (reaching forward), MAS items 3 (sitting balance) and 5 (walking) and TUG.

Study IV: Descriptive statistics were used to summarise demographic, stroke and baseline characteristics. All analyses were performed on an intention-to-treat basis. Means, medians and SD were calculated for each clinical test. A general linear model, with a univariate ANOVA was performed, using baseline to one year change as dependent variable on each of the scores of MAS, BI, and grip strength, with treatment group as a primary factor and age and gender as covariates. In addition, differences in improvement were calculated for total score on MAS, BI and grip strength and analysed in the same manner. A subgroup analysis of the dichotomised values of the Motor Assessment Scale and Barthel Index of Activities of Daily Living was also performed.

4.3.4 Ethical considerations

The studies were all approved by the Regional Committee of Medical Research Ethics of Norway. Informed consent was given by all participants through methods approved by the same Committee. Oral and written information about the studies was given.

5   Results

The main results of the studies are presented in papers I-IV.

5.1 Study I

Patients treated according to the Motor Relearning Programme (71) stayed fewer days in hospital than those treated by the Bobath approach (148) (mean number of days 21 versus 34, p=0.008). Both groups improved their scores in MAS (181) and SMES (182), but the improvement in motor function was significantly better in the MRP group (Table 2). The two groups improved in BI (183) scores but there were no significant differences between the groups. However, there was a significant difference in the BI subscores bladder (p=0.01), bowel (p=0.004), and independence in toilet situations (p=0.02), in favour of the MRP group. Women treated by MRP improved more than women treated by Bobath method. There were no differences between the groups in the life quality test (NHP) (184), use of assistive devices or accommodation after discharge from the hospital.

Table 2: Study I: Total scores of Motor Assessment Scale (MAS), Södring Motor Evaluation Scale (SMES) and Barthel Index of ADL (BI) on three test occasions in two different groups, the Motor Relearning Programme group (MRP) and the Bobath training group, mean/median, SD and p values. Maximal points for each test within brackets.

	MRP (n = 33)			Bobath (n = 28)			p values, repeated measurements, between groups
	3 days	2 weeks	3 months	3 days	2 weeks	3 months	
Number of patients	33	30	29	28	27	24	
MAS (48)	24/29	32/40	37/42	19/20	23/25	33/39	0.002
SD	14	15	12	15	16	15	
SMES 1 (20)	12/13	15/16	17/20	11/12	14/16	16/19	0.21
SD	5	6	5	5	6	6	
SMES 2 (70)	47/51	58/65	65/76	39/35	48/51	58/65	0.02
SD	19	23	21	23	24	23	
SMES 3 (60)	20/19	32/37	41/44	18/15	30/32	39/48	0.51
SD	16	20	18	18	21	21	
BI (100)	56/60		83/95	46/55		72/88	0.19

5.2 Study II

Both groups showed a decrease in motor function, postural control and ADL at one and four years, leaving many of the patients dependent and with a risk of falling (Table 3). Quality of Life had increased but was still low in comparison with that of healthy persons of similar age. Patients in both groups continued to live at home to a great extent, but were dependent on help from relatives or the community services. Physiotherapy as a follow-up service was seldom used. The choice of initial physiotherapy approach did not seem to have any influence on the patients' ability to cope in the long run.

Table 3 Outcomes for the Motor Relearning Programme (MRP) and Bobath groups measured on three occasions after stroke. Mean/median values and SD are given. MAS =Motor Assessment scale; SMES = Södring Motor Evaluation scale; BI = Barthel Index of ADL: NHP = Nottingham Health Profile. Maximal scores for each test are given within brackets.

	MRP (n = 33)			**Bobath** (n=28)		
	3 months	1 year	4 years	3 months	1 year	4 years
Number of patients (n)						
	29	27	21	24	21	16
Deaths (n)	4	6	12	4	7	12
MAS (48)	37/42	30/37	21/26	33/39	27/36	19/17
SD	12	18	21	15	20	20
SMES 1 (20)	17/20	13/16	9/12	16/19	12/16	8/9
SD	5	7	9	6	8	9
SMES 2 (60)	67/76	52/64	33/18	58/65	47/72	32/22
SD	21	31	35	23	36	22
SMES 3 (70)	41/44	32/36	22/21	39/48	31/35	21/17
SD	18	23	24	21	25	24
BI (100)	83/95	68/95	45/60	72/88	57/75	42/40
SD	25	41	44	34	43	44
NHP (100)	22/19	17/15	20/21	24/21	13/11	16/15
SD	18	16	15	21	12	11
Living at home	17	20	13	13	14	13

5.3 Study III

On admission 41 of the 57 patients were able to walk to some extent, whereas on discharge all 57 could walk. Twenty-seven patients were discharged to their own home, 19 to rehabilitation units and 11 to nursing homes (short-term).

The median score of BI (183) was 75 (Inter Quartile Range (IQR) = 70) on admission and 90, (IQR = 45) on discharge. The results on admission and at discharge are presented in Table 4. The patients with stroke improved significantly both in gait velocity, from 0.7 to 0.8 m/s, and in 6 minutes' walking distance, from 234 to 294 m, between admission and discharge. Significant improvements were also noted for scores of MAS (181) item 3 (sitting balance), MAS item 5 (walking), BBS (185) item 6 (standing with feet together, blindfolded) and BBS item 8 (reaching distance). The mean score for reaching distance as measured with BBS item 8 was around 3, representing a mean reaching distance of 12-15 cm (Table 4).

Sixteen of 57 patients were unable to perform TUG (187) on admission, compared with five at discharge. The mean value for TUG (n = 41) was 16.4 s on admission and 11.1 s at discharge (n = 41) (Table 4). This improvement was significant (p<0.001) and had a high correlation with gait velocity and gait distance (r_s = 0.71 / - 0.71).

Table 4: Mean values and standard deviation of 6-minute walk test, Motor Assessment Scale (MAS) items 3 (sitting balance) and 5 (walking), Berg Balance Scale (BBS) items 6 (standing balance) and 8 (reaching), and Timed Up-and-Go (TUG) in stroke patients on admission to and at discharge from a stroke unit.

	Admission n = 57	Discharge n = 57	p values between admission-discharge
Distance in 6 minutes (m)	234 (208)	294 (198)	p<0.001
Gait velocity (m/s)	0.7 (0.5)	0.8 (0.5)	p<0.001
MAS item 3 (max score 6)	4.4 (2.0)	5.1 (1.5)	p<0.001
MAS item 5 (max score 6)	3.5 (2.5)	4.1 (2.0)	p<0.001
BBS item 6 (max score 4)	2.6 (1.9)	3.4 (1.3)	p<0.001
BBS item 8 (max score 4)	2.0 (1.8)	2.6 (1.5)	p<0.001
TUG (s) n=41	16.4 (14.0)	11.1 (24.8)	p<0.001

Correlation coefficients at test 1 between 6 MWT (186) and the balance measures MAS items 3 and 5, and BBS items 6 and 8, were between 0.75 and 0.82 (Table 5). The same correlations were somewhat lower (0.56 – 0.67) at discharge. The correlation coefficients between TUG and 6MWT, for those who were able to perform at both tests, (n = 41), were high ($r_s = -0.80 / -0.73$).

Table 5 Spearman's rank correlation coefficients between 6- Minute Walk Test (6 MWT) and Motor assessment (MAS) items 3 and 5, Berg Balance Scale (BBS) items 6 and 8 and Timed Up-and-Go (TUG) at admission and discharge in 57 patients with stroke.

	6MWT Admission		6MWT Discharge	
	r	p value	r	p value
MAS item 3 (sitting balance)	0.75	< 0.001	0.56	<0.001
MAS item 5 (walking)	0.81	< 0.001	0.67	< 0.001
BBS item 6 (standing, blindfolded)	0.53	< 0.001	0.47	= 0.001
BBS item 8 (reaching)	0.82	< 0.001	0.60	< 0.001
TUG **(n=41)**	-0.80	< 0.001	-0.73	< 0.001

A regression analysis with all variables included yielded an adjusted R^2 of 0.85 on admission and 0.76 at discharge, showing a strong relationship between gait velocity and all balance measures together (Table 6). In the stepwise regression analysis MAS item 5 (walking) ($p<0.01$) was found to be the strongest explanatory factor for gait velocity. When MAS item 5 (walking) was removed, TUG ($p<0.001$), MAS item 3 ($p<0.01$) (sitting balance) and BBS item 8 ($p<0.03$) (reaching distance) were the strongest explanatory factors on admission, with an adjusted R^2 of 0.83. At discharge, the strongest explanatory factors were TUG ($p = 0.02$), MAS item 3 ($p<0.001$), BBS item 8 ($p<0.001$) (reaching distance), with an adjusted R^2 of 0.73.

Table 6: Regression analysis showing the association between gait velocity and the independent variables Motor Assessment Scale (MAS) 3 (sitting balance), Berg Balance Scale (BBS) 6 (standing blindfolded), BBS 8 (reaching distance) and Timed Up-and-Go (TUG) test on admission (Test 1) and discharge (Test 2).

Variables	Beta	SE	p values
Test 1			
MAS 3	0.16	0.03	0.01
BBS 6	-0.04	0.03	0.73
BBS 8	0.64	0.03	0.03
TUG	-0.24	0.003	0.001
Test 2			
MAS 3	0.37	0.04	0.001
BBS 6	-0.13	0.04	0.33
BBS 8	0.58	0.04	0.001
TUG	-0.17	0.001	0.02

Note: Test 1, adjusted $R^2 = 0.85$; test 2, $R^2 = 0.76$

There is a strong relationship between walking and balance, both dynamic and static in the acute rehabilitation of patients with stroke, indicating that static and dynamic balance needs to be addressed equally in the early rehabilitation of stroke patients, and is closely related to task, e.g. walking, getting up from a chair, turning, and reaching, and cannot be regarded as separate from the task.

5.4 Study IV

Both groups improved significantly in motor function (MAS) (181), activities of daily living (BI) (183) and grip strength (vigorimeter) (188) from admission to three months post-stroke. Between the three-month and six–month follow-up this improvement stabilised and there were no significant further improvements in either of the groups. At one year of follow-up there was a tendency to a reduction of performance in MAS and BI in both groups, whereas grip strength still seemed to be improving.

There were significant differences in degrees of improvement from admission to discharge, in favour of the intensive exercise group, regarding the MAS total score and sub-scores for turning in bed, standing up, upper extremity function and hand function, and also for the BI total score and sub-scores for dressing, transfer from bed to chair, walking capacity, and walking up and down stairs (Table 7). There were also significant group differences in improvement of grip strength in the paretic hand from the three- to six-month follow-up, and of the MAS total scores from the six-month to the one-year follow-up (Table 7).

The mean motor function at baseline, as assessed by MAS, was higher in the regular exercise group (m=31.4) than in the intensive exercise group (m=26.7). The regular exercise group also had higher baseline values for activities of daily living, as measured by BI (regular exercise group m=66; intensive exercise group m=56.6) and for grip strength, as assessed with the vigorimeter (regular exercise group 0.41 and 0.65 kp (bar); intensive exercise group 0.37 and 0.55 kp (bar). The differences were not significant, however.

The patients were also divided into those with lower MAS scores (0 – 35) and those with higher scores (36 - 48) and the results confirmed the observed differences between the two exercise groups, although they were not significant. Fifty-four per cent of the patients in the intensive exercise group and 45 % of those in the regular exercise group scored low on admission. This difference had levelled out at discharge, when 40 % and 42 %, respectively, scored low. At the three-month follow-up the levelling had ceased and 38 % in the intensive exercise group versus 30 % in the regular exercise group had low scores. At the one-year follow-up 34 % of the intensive exercise group patients and 19 % of those in the regular exercise group had low scores. None of these differences were significant, however.

The same development was observed regarding activities of daily living when the scores were divided into low scores of 0 – 59 and high scores of 60 – 100 for analysis. At discharge, 26 % in the intensive exercise group and 28 % in the regular exercise group scored low on the BI. At the one-year follow-up 28 % of the intensive exercise group and 10 % of the regular exercise group had low scores. None of these differences were significant.

The patients in both groups were highly motivated for training and 25 patients in the intensive exercise group (71 %) and 26 patients in the regular exercise group (65 %) stated spontaneously on the test occasions that they found the exercises vital for their function and well-being. Compliance to the training programmes was high in 28 patients (80 %) in the intensive exercise group and in 31 patients (78 %) in the regular exercise group. The intensity of the programme was high in both groups, with a tendency to therapeutically steered training in the intensive exercise group and more self-initiated training in the regular exercise group.

Between the three-month and the 12-month follow-up the mean number of occasions of supervised exercise in the intensive exercise group was 2.1 times per week and in the regular exercise group 2.2 times per week. This amounts to approximately 40 weeks of exercise per year in both groups, which represents the 80 hours we initially aimed at in the intensive exercise group.

All patients included in the study came from their own homes in the local communities when admitted to the hospital. At discharge 15 out of 32 patients in the intensive exercise group and 19 out of 35 in the regular exercise group were discharged to their own homes, and at the one-year follow-up 24 and 29 patients in these two groups, respectively, were living at home. There were no significant differences in this respect.

There was a significant difference in the length of stay at the acute hospital. The mean stay of the patients in the intensive exercise group was 22 days, as compared to 16 days in the regular exercise group ($p = 0.03$).

The patients of the intensive exercise group were receiving more help from relatives and the community on all test occasions. These differences were significant only at one year of follow-up ($p = 0.04$).

Pain was being experienced by 15 of the intensive exercise group patients and by 13 of the patients in the regular exercise group at the end of the one-year follow-up period. Three patients in the intensive exercise group and one in the regular exercise group reported having had a fall during the whole period.

Thus, the overall results of this study were positive, indicating that a more intensive follow-up programme during the first year after stroke is highly favourable.

Table 7: The mean difference in improvement of total scores, between different test occasions, for the Motor Assessment Scale (MAS), Barthel ADL Index (BI) and grip strength measured in bar in the paretic and non-paretic hand, with p values for significant differences between the groups. adm. = admission; dis. = discharge; * p < 0.05

	Intervention group n=35	Regular training group n=40	p values
MAS adm – dis	7.5	1.7	0.01*
MAS dis – 3 months	2.2	4.6	0.54
MAS 3 – 6 months	1.5	0.9	0.61
MAS 6 months -1 year	-1.2	1.4	0.02*
BI adm – dis	18.9	9.8	0.04*
BI dis – 3 months	7.46	11.8	0.91
BI 3 – 6 months	1.54	3.6	0.44
BI 6 months – 1 year	-3.7	-3.5	0.71
Grip strength paretic hand adm - dis	0.03	0.07	0.67
Grip strength paretic hand dis – 3 months	0.06	0.06	0.86
Grip strength paretic hand 3-6 months	0.14	0.01	0.04*
Grip strength paretic hand 6 months- 1 year	0.08	0.12	0.16
Grip strength non-paretic hand adm – dis	0.07	0.08	0.76
Grip strength non-paretic hand dis – 3 months	0.06	0.06	0.90
Grip strength non-paretic hand 3-6 months	0.09	0.02	0.11
Grip strength non-paretic hand 6 months – 1 year	0.1	0.18	0.61

6 General discussion

6.1 Design

Studies I, II and IV were designed as experimental, longitudinal, randomised, controlled stratified trials. The process of randomisation was performed in the same way in all three studies. Patients were randomised to one of two different groups by a person not involved with the patients or the treatment in the ward. The randomisation periods, however, were different. In studies I and II randomisation took place immediately after the diagnosis was verified, while in study IV it was carried out at discharge from the acute hospital.

The protocol was sealed for three months in studies I and II, and for 1.5 years in study IV. The studies were double-blind intention-to-treat trials. Neither the investigator nor the patients knew to which group they were allocated in studies I and IV. In study II the intervention ceased after approximately three months, at the same time as the blinding was broken.

In clinical studies the difficulty in being blinded without contamination can be a problem. In all our studies the test person was not active in the clinic or the hospital, which should have made him/her person "neutral". The patients were not informed about what type of exercise/treatment they were given, so they did not know the "name" of their therapy or that they had been placed in any special group. The therapists leading the exercises were only engaged in one type of exercise in the whole period, so there was no mixing of exercise protocols. In this respect contamination of blinding procedures was kept to a minimum and we have chosen to call it double-blind. This statement is perhaps debatable and it may be argued that in a strict sense, the studies were single-blind, since we have no assurance that the patients did not find out that they were placed in one or the other group.

Study III was a non-experimental study with no intervention and no group allocation, although the same procedures of inclusion and exclusion criteria were followed.
On all test occasions the assessor was a well experienced clinical physiotherapist, well acquainted with the tests, which would minimise any violation of intra-rater reliability. In the case of the self-report the questions were asked verbally. So that the patients could familiarise themselves with the content of the self-reported test, they were given the text before the structured interview.

6.2 Methods

6.2.1 Patient selection

Patients were selected on the general basis of the stroke population admitted to the stroke unit at a general hospital on, two different occasions in the periods 1996 – 1997 (studies I and II) and 2003-2004 (studies III and IV), in order to describe the effects of physiotherapy in the short- and long-term perspectives.

In order to get a representative stroke population, it was vital to include only first-time-ever stroke patients. Furthermore, the inclusion and exclusion criteria were the same in all studies, so that the results could be considered comparable (I-IV). This procedure should have ensured that the populations were as homogeneous as possible, considering the facts that the time intervals differed and that persons suffering from stroke in general are to be considered a heterogeneous population. On the other hand, the fact that the patients were recruited at the same local hospital on both occasions might limit the generalisation of the results to this particular local area of the world.

Inclusion criteria were first-time-ever stroke with neurological signs, verified clinically and by computed tomography, and voluntary participation. It was important that all patients should have as equal a start as possible that the differences in impairments and disabilities were equally and randomly distributed in both groups. This procedure would reduce the variability between the patients and the groups.

In order to evaluate different approaches and intensities of physiotherapy, the persons treated needed to have some neurological deficits and verification by CT of that these deficits were actually due to a stroke and not to another medical condition.

Exclusion criteria were more than one stroke incident, stroke to the brain stem or cerebellum, subarachnoid haemorrhage and tumours of the brain, as all these conditions have a different pattern of recovery compared with that in patients with first-time stroke. Stroke patients with other severe medical conditions were also excluded, since these might seriously affect the patient's activity level in the rehabilitation period and this again might be a reason for a patient not being able to participate in the programmes, compromising compliance. These conditions might also have a different recovery pattern compared with stroke.

In general approximately 250 – 300 patients per year are admitted to the local hospital with a final diagnosis of stroke. On the basis of estimates from our earlier studies (124, 144) we needed a total of 60 -70 patients with first-time-ever stroke to detect a difference in motor function with a significance level of 0.05 and a power of 80 %.

It was vital that patients were consecutively included in the trial as soon as they were admitted to the hospital if they fulfilled the inclusion criteria, in order to get that number of patients. This was also a practical arrangement, planned so that the studies would be concluded within a reasonable time limit and with as few drop-outs as possible. It was the aim that the study populations should be considered representative and comparable to the general stroke population admitted to the stroke unit at any time.

6.2.2 Outcome measures

Outcome measures and tests were chosen to allow evaluation of the effectiveness of different treatment approaches as relevantly as possible. In studies I and II it was important that motor function should be measured as objectively as possible in order to capture possible strengths of the two approaches; Bobath and Motor Relearning Programme. For that purpose two different motor evaluations were incorporated in the tests, namely MAS (181), with its functional level, and SMES (182), with its test of quality of movement in parts 1 and 2. If functional improvements were "compensatory", in the respect that the patients were encouraged to use his/her good side in order to go through with the task, this would be captured and unmasked by SMES, which would evaluate quality of movement to a higher degree than MAS, and thus capture one of the main goals of normal movement to which the Bobath method aspires. MAS, on the other hand would capture the functional aspects of movement to a higher degree than SMES, and as was hypothesised, would be able to link improvement to the ICF disability level. The two different evaluations of motor control (MAS and SMES) could also, if improvements were found, capture different "gains" both in function and in the quality of motor performance. It could be hypothesised that one of the approaches might have a more pronounced long-term impact than the other and that the result of this impact might not become evident until the three- month or one-year follow-up. In order to test this hypothesis, it was important to explore motor function from both functional ("quantity") and quality points of view.

It was also important to target different levels of ICIDH / ICF (79), in order to elucidate the question whether and how the two different physiotherapy interventions had an impact on one or more levels. It has been hypothesised, and has also been a general belief in therapy, that improving function on the impairment level, e.g. by increasing strength through exercise, will automatically transfer to activities such as improved gait. That is, that this increased function on the impairment level will also contribute to a higher degree of activity and participation e.g. increased P- and I-ADL or a better quality of life (216). In order to test

44

this belief, the Barthel Index of Activities of Daily Living (183) was chosen to monitor activities in combination with impairments, tested with SMES (182). BI is a frequently used ADL instrument in the clinic and in stroke trials (183,192).

At the three-month, one-year and four-year follow-ups, a health-related quality of life test (NHP) was added in studies I and II to represent ICF´s participation level (184, 211-212). This test was different from MAS (181), SMES (182) and BI (183), since it was the patient's own evaluation of health and function that was in focus, and not the performance evaluated by the therapist according to a standardised test. It became apparent that patients´ evaluation of their function and health differed from the results of the performance-based assessments, a finding which prompted us to conduct a study where we compared self perceived and performance-based evaluations (217). The outcome of that study (217) confirmed previous results indicating that NHP (184) measures other values than are assessed in the motor function tests (181-183). From the aspect of a disablement process model (ICF / Nagi) (79, 218) it could be argued that performance-based tests reflect functional limitations and the self-reported tests reflect disability (219-221). This would imply that self-reported tests indicate the level of performance of a task in the usual daily circumstances and performance-based measures show how well an individual can carry out a task in a clinical environment (219).

In study III the focus was on gait capacity and its relation to balance, both static and dynamic, and the measurements should reflect the capacity to walk a reasonably long distance, and the capacity to walk fast. On admission to and discharge from the acute stroke unit, all patients were tested with the 6MWT (gait velocity and distance) (186), MAS (181), items 3 (sitting balance) and 5 (walking), BBS (185), items 6 (standing blindfolded) and 8 (reaching forward, TUG (187) and BI (P-ADL) (183). The 6MWT was ideal, that both distance and ability to maintain a high velocity during a relatively long period were tested. At the same time the patient's ability to assess his/her own capability to carry out the 6MWT at the speed chosen was also tested. In a way, endurance, motor function and coping skill were tested at the same time (195, 200). Walking capacity was also tested by MAS, subscale 5, and BI, subscale 9, but the distance was shorter. The balance measures in this study were chosen to mirror dynamic and static balance, since the purpose of the study was to test the hypotheses that balance, both static and dynamic, is related to task and is equally important to address in the rehabilitation of acute stroke.

The outcome measures in study IV were chosen to reflect the three different levels of WHO´s ICF (79), impairments, activity and participation, by common clinical measures used in stroke rehabilitation. The purpose of the study was to evaluate two different exercise programmes in the post-stroke rehabilitation of patients with first-ever stroke over a period of one year and if possible to relate this to impairment, activity and participation according to ICF.

Measurements on the impairment level, in the same study, were grip strength and the Modified Ashworth Scale (222), which measures spasticity (results not presented in this thesis). Grip strength is an indicator of overall muscle strength (223). Grip strength is also associated with ADL (224) and can be said to represent motor function on the impairment level (225). Increased tone and /or spasticity have been one of the main therapeutic aims in physiotherapy for many years. It has been argued that an increased exercise load might increase tone; for this reason strength training and maximal load principles in general have been avoided by therapists (148). In order to evaluate the two exercise programmes from all angles of motor function in the present studies, it was vital to incorporate a measurement of tone, in this case the Modified Ashworth Scale, since the principles of maximal load were recommended in one of the exercise groups in study IV (222). However, there is some controversy as to which component of muscle function the scale is measuring, and thus its validity as a measure of spasticity or muscle tone is unclear (226-227). The Modified Ashworth Scale has been the most widely used test of spasticity in clinical practice. In recent years, however, the Tardieu scale has been reintroduced (228), and some authors consider this test to be a more valid clinical tool, since it differentiates spasticity from contracture (229). In our study, however, it was important to know whether the tone increased or not and whether this could be related to any of the interventions. The component responsible for a possible increase; hyperactive reflexes or contracture, was in this case of minor consequence.

Measurements on the activity level in study IV were MAS (181), BI (183), 6MWT (186), TUG (187) and BBS (185), which give information on motor function and activity, ADL, gait velocity and distance, balance and mobility, all of which are vital functions not only in themselves but also in relation to one another.

Finally, measurements on the participation level were The Duke Older Americans Resources and Service Procedures (OARS), the Multidimensional Functional assessment of Older Adults by Fillenbaum (216)(not presented in this thesis) and NHP (184). Fillenbaum's test is related to I-ADL, and NHP concerns health-related quality of life. These two measurements reflect different aspects of participation and can be related to different measures on the impairment and activity levels.

46

6.2.3 Statistical approach

Descriptive statistics were used to present data in all studies summarised in this thesis. This is a simple way to present data and they are also easy to read (260).

The level of significance in all studies was set to 5 %, an arbitrary level set by the researcher. A power analysis was made in preparation for studies I and IV in order to correctly identify any differences between the groups. The power of a test can be influenced by sample size, effect size and alpha level (significance level, e.g. 0.05 or 0.01). It has been suggested that when small group sizes are involved it may be necessary to adjust the alpha level to compensate, for example by having a cut-off of 0.10 or 0.15, rather than the traditional 0.05 level (261).

In studies I and II Student's t-test was used (MAS, BI) for comparing the mean scores of two different groups. The analyses were also run with a non-parametric Mann-Whitney test, but since the results were similar the parametric statistics was kept according to "the central limit theorem" (260). We also made use of ANOVA for repeated measurements with a Bonferroni correction, to see if there was a difference between the two groups in terms of effectiveness in enhancing motor function, ADL and quality of life. A further aim was to see if this change in performance was different in the two groups over the three time periods. The Bonferroni adjustment is one way to control for Type I error, by dividing the normal alpha value, 0.05, by the number of tests performed. A Mann-Whitney non-parametric test was conducted on the Nottingham Health Profile and continuous measures between the groups, i.e. gender differences, use of assistive devices, and destination after discharge. The Friedman test, the non-parametric alternative to the repeated measurements, was used for analysing NHP over time.

In study III we also made use of a multiple linear regression analysis to estimate the association between the dependent variable gait velocity and five independent variables: MAS 5 and 3, BBS 6 and 8, and TUG. A multiple regression analysis is based on the assumptions of normal distribution and a linear relationship between the dependent and each independent variable. The multicollinarity problem should also be assessed. This refers to a situation where two or more independent variables are highly correlated and implies the inclusion of two or more redundant variables in the analysis. MAS 5 was excluded in our model because of collinearity. To test for collinearity, the variance of inflation factor (VIF) and the Tolerance value (261-262) were used. The distribution of the residuals was examined for normality using the Kolmogorov-Smirnov test.

In study IV we used a general linear model, with a univariate ANOVA and Bonferroni correction on each of the scores of MAS, BI and grip strength with treatment group as primary factor and gender as covariate. The advantage of this two-way design is that we can test the main effect of each independent variable and also explore the possibility of an interaction effect. We also used the mixed model analysis when modelling the change over time with the variables group, time for test and scores of MAS, BI and grip strength respectively. Main effects and all two-way interactions were included in the model. The mixed model analysis did not add more information and we have therefore reported the results from the original General Linear Model (GLM).

6.3 Discussion - Results

6.3.1 Bobath or Motor Relearning Programme? (study I)

This study was the first to show a difference, related to length of stay and motor function in first-ever-stroke patients, between two physiotherapy approaches in the rehabilitation of acute stroke where all other aspects of the treatment programme were kept alike for all patients.

The study focused on two different motor control theories that are dominant within physiotherapy and stroke rehabilitation (92). The programmes reflecting two different motor control theories, the Bobath concept (148), which can be considered to be based on the reflex-hierarchy theory (92, 148) and the Motor Relearning Programme (MRP) (84), based on a systems approach (92, 84). We specified the physiotherapy treatments reflecting the two theories specified in two different manuals, which formed guidelines for the treatment, which in study I was carried out by two different teams of physiotherapists during the acute stage at the stroke unit and the following sub-acute rehabilitation period (attachments 1-4). The MRP guidelines were based on a textbook by Carr & Shepherd (84) and were commented on by Carr and Shepherd by correspondence (attachment 2). The Bobath guidelines were based on a book by Bertha and Karel Bobath (148) and on the physiotherapists' perception of the programmes as they had experienced them from the Bobath courses (attachment 3). In conjunction with these guidelines, talks, workshops and discussions on the practice of the MRP and Bobath methods formed the training and practice in the two groups. The physiotherapists treating the MRP group did this exclusively and the same applied to the physiotherapists who treated the Bobath group. All physiotherapists were experienced and had a minimum of 10 years´ practice.

The result of this study indicated that physiotherapy with the MRP approach was preferable to that following the Bobath concept in the acute rehabilitation of stroke patients. That is, a systems approach, in this case MRP, which defines movement as an interaction between the individual, the task and the environment and sees movement as the result of a dynamic interplay between perceptual, cognitive and action systems (84, 92), was more beneficial than a reflex-hierarchical approach, as represented by the Bobath treatment, where "normal movement" is facilitated and "abnormal movement", associated reactions and spasticity are inhibited (148).

The criticism and discussion around this study have been related to the authors´ interpretation of the Bobath concept and to whether or not the Bobath method is a reflex-hierarchical method or not. The most ardent critics of the study consider that the Bobath concept has changed and that it is now a programme based on a systems approach, and claim that there are no differences between the methods. This might be the case and may also explain why recent studies have had difficulty in reproducing our results (230).

However, this is not in conformity with the published literature and with the official side of the International Bobath Instructors Training Association (IBITA) (231), presenting the Bobath concept. The presented therapy is based on the same "normal movement", the proximal key components shoulders and hips, "handling of the patient", and inhibiting of associated reactions and spasticity as presented by the Bobaths originally (148), but now with references to recent research and systems approach theories. This give reason to believe that the common practice is the same as ever, but those explanatory motor control theories have been changed to suit recent research. If this is the case, this might lead to confusion in clinical practice, since motor control theories and clinical practice operate on different levels and the treatment protocols are not identical.

This indicates the importance of our study, where therapeutic input has to be defined in accordance with theories of motor control (92, 139) and a model of disablement (92, 139). In order to change the basis of clinical practice from one motor control theory to another, one has to be aware of what explanatory models are being used in order to redirect into something else (138-139). Physiotherapy should be based on the *"clinical decision-making process"*, which includes gathering information, which is essential for developing a plan of care, that is consistent with the problems and needs of the patient (92). This in turn is based on *"hypothesis-oriented clinical practice"*, which means systematical testing of assumptions about the nature and cause of motor control problems and reflects the theories of a clinician about the cause and nature of function and dysfunction in patients with neurological disease (92). It is therefore of vital importance to describe what is being done in clinical practice in terms of exercises, repetitions, intensity, frequency and length of exercise classes and to whom it is done and their age, gender and health problems, in order to evaluate the same exercises in the light of the hypothesis and also to place the assessment and plan of treatment in the framework of the disablement model, for example WHO´s ICF (79).

In our study we tested the hypothesis of two motor control theories; the systems approach versus the reflex-hierarchical concept. We evaluated the results within the frame of ICF and found that a programme based on the systems approach was beneficial. The result of our study suggests that clinical practice should be based on the *clinical decision-making process* and that task-oriented physiotherapy should be chosen in preference to physiotherapy that aims to prevent spasticity and associated reactions and to stabilise the trunk and head in order to prepare the patient with stroke for exercises.

Handling patients with stroke in accordance with specified theories of motor control, "a global aspect", has been and is today a driving force in physiotherapy and stroke rehabilitation (84, 92, 148). Our study I was the first to test this global aspect in acute stroke rehabilitation and also seems to have led to the adoption of a systems approach. The recommendations from Cochrane reviews are also clear: "There is a need for high quality randomised trials and systematic reviews to determine the efficacy of clearly described individual techniques and task-specific treatments" (167).

The National Board of Health and Welfare in Sweden recommends task-oriented therapy in the acute treatment of patients with stroke (level 3 on a range from 1-10) and does not recommend therapies that are not based on the task-oriented approach, such as Bobath and PNF because of lack of evidence (18). The Ottawa panel (20) also found good evidence for task-oriented therapy; the panel concludes that such therapy should be strongly recommended in the rehabilitation of stroke patients and agrees with other clinical guidelines which do not to recommend the use of the Bobath approach at large.

6.3.2 Bobath or Motor Relearning Programme? A follow-up (study II)

The main findings in this study were a high mortality rate and a decrease in function in the survivors one and four years after stroke, irrespective of the physiotherapy given during the primary rehabilitation. The decrease in function was more pronounced than in the average population of old people (232). The decline in motor function and ADL was compensated by help from relatives and community–based services. Despite this reduction of motor and ADL function, the health-related quality of life, as measured by NHP (184), was reportedly better than at three months of follow-up, but was low compared with that of healthy counterparts (232-234).

In general the patients received little or no physiotherapy after the first rehabilitation period. This finding was in sharp contrast to the initial stroke care received by the patients. The lack of follow-up treatment, in combination with the increased burden on the relatives, was also contradictory to the increased health-related quality of life, as measured by NHP (184), which was self-reported. It seemed as if the performance-based and the self-reported assessments measured different aspects, as we also have observed in another study (217).

However, if in Norway a doctor refers a patient with a diagnosis of stroke to a physiotherapist, the patient have a "right" to 80 hours´ physiotherapy free of charge in the community per year. It was puzzling that this possibility was not utilised to a greater extent. It might be speculated whether the reason for this could be an expectation that the interventions in the acute stage would carry over in the longer perspective? Or was it possibly expected that interventions in the acute rehabilitation stage would lead to a higher activity level auto-matically and indirectly contribute to higher participation and thus would keep the body functioning on "all levels"?

Our follow-up made it quite clear that physiotherapy in the acute stroke unit / acute rehabilitation did not carry over in relation to time, irrespective of what kind of physiotherapy - MRP (84) or Bobath (148) - the patient had received during the initial stage.
The discrepancy between the results of the health-related quality of life test and the motor and ADL function tests at one year led to study IV.

6.3.3 The relation between gait velocity and static and dynamic balance in the early rehabilitation of patients with acute stroke (study III)

The most important finding in this study was that gait, measured with 6MWT (196-198) was equally related to static and dynamic balance in the very early stage after an acute stroke. The strong relationship between static balance and gait velocity on admission indicates a need for enhancement of stability at this early stage in stroke patients (235-238). On the other hand the relationship between gait velocity and dynamic balance indicates that dynamic balance, also, is related to gait velocity at this early stage of recovery (237). The clinical implication being that balance, both static and dynamic, should be equally addressed at the early rehabilitation stage, and that balance, both static and dynamic, is related to task, e.g. walking, getting up

51

from a chair, turning, and reaching, and cannot be regarded as separate from the task (40, 239).

Improved dynamic balance was also a highly explanatory factor of increased gait velocity. The resemblance of tasks, requiring cognitive, sensory and visual coordination, is one factor connecting the two. Another is improved muscular function and presumably improved strategies for accomplishing the task (40, 115, 239-243). From a clinical point of view, the improvements are fairly moderate compared to values in healthy older people of corresponding age, indicating dependence on assistive devices (244). Considering the fact that many of the patients with stroke are sent home at this point of rehabilitation, this might indicate a risk of falls and/or inactivity because of limited function, and huge costs in energy when performing daily activities.

In many ways this study confirms the results of study I (144), and supports a systems approach. Movement is dependent on an interaction between the individual, the task and the environment, where movement is the result of a dynamic interplay between perceptual, cognitive and action systems (92). Walking capacity and gait velocity are related to balance, both dynamic and static. In order to address walking capacity in the acute stage of stroke rehabilitation, static balance cannot be addressed alone in a hierarchical fashion, "stability before mobility", but the task walking need to addressed at the same time as task-related static and dynamic balance components.

6.3.4 Stroke patients and long-term training: is it worthwhile? A randomised comparison of two different training strategies after rehabilitation (study IV)

This study is, to our knowledge, the first randomised controlled trial in which an intensive exercise programme is compared with regular treatment in patients with first-time-ever stroke during the first year after the period in the acute stroke unit. Other similar studies have concerned patients with chronic stroke (161, 164, 166, 249-254) and patients with mixed first- and second-time stroke (77, 161,164, 166, 249 - 250, 252 -254) with interventions for shorter periods. The improved function in these studies could also be seen as a reduction of secondary complications and inactivity after stroke and not as prolonged recovery after stroke. The benefit of treating a group of patients with first-time stroke for a longer period, such as one year as in our study, is that the secondary complications in connection with inactivity are minimised. The improvement and maintenance of function can then be attributable to the spontaneous recovery and rehabilitation.

Our main findings were that the improvements in motor function, activities of daily living and grip strength during the acute rehabilitation period continued and were maintained during the first year after stroke. These observations were made in both the intensive exercise group and regular exercise group, contrary to our hypothesis. However, the exercise levels were high in both groups in this study, higher in the regular-exercise group than anticipated from earlier experience (124). This was unintentional, but probably due to high motivation on the part of all participants regardless of their group allocation. We believe that this high motivation was triggered by the test occasions and regular contact with a physiotherapist, leading to higher exercise levels in the regular exercise group, identical to those of the intensive exercise group. In this study, the improvements in MAS (181) and BI (183) scores, in both groups, were larger at three months and one year than were found in a previous follow-up study of stroke patients who received little or no treatment in the after-stroke period (124). Such improvements and the maintenance of motor function, activities of daily living and grip strength in patients with first-time-ever stroke have not, to our knowledge, been demonstrated in any other study. In our opinion, these positive results are due to the regular exercise programmes and the regular follow-ups three, six and twelve months following the acute stroke.

We did not find any significant differences in motor function, activities of daily living or grip strength between the intensive exercise and regular exercise group on any test occasion. This might be explained by several factors. One is that the motor function and activities of daily living were slightly better in the regular exercise group than in the intensive exercise group at the first test on admission. This difference should not, however, have had an impact on the patients' reactions to the rehabilitative input, since even the most severely affected patients may experience meaningful improvement during early rehabilitation (37, 55, 255-258).

Regarding the different degrees of improvement in the two groups, there were significantly greater improvements in the intensive exercise group in the total MAS score and the total BI score during the first rehabilitation period between admission and discharge (Table 7). Grip strength of the paretic hand showed the same tendency between the three- and six-month tests (Table 7). It might seem that the poorer function in the intensive exercise group on admission was compensated by a more sensitive and rapid reaction to therapy in the early rehabilitation stage.

The training levels, compliance and motivation were equally high in the two groups. There was no difference in training habits or follow-ups between the groups on any of the test occasions (Table 5). The intensive training that was compulsory in the intensive exercise group was compensated by an extensive self-training programme in the regular exercise group. This result was somewhat surprising. Our earlier study had revealed little or no physical activity in the first year after stroke (124). This high compliance and training could have been triggered by the regular test occasions, which all patients of both groups were informed would take place three months, six months and one year after the stroke. The test occasions in themselves were strong motivators for training and seemed to make the participants, irrespective of group allocation, aware of their own need for exercise. This supportive role of supervision or of inclusion in a social group has also been noted in a study by Olney et al (259). The result can also be compared with findings in similar studies where social support, defined as "the experience of information that one is loved and cared for, valued and esteemed and able to count on others should the need arise" (245), has resulted in a sense of control which has improved the individual's ability to cope with stress (131, 246-247)

One of the weaknesses of study IV is the fact that for different reasons the two groups were equally active in doing physical exercises. We did not have a true control with which to compare our findings. However, the results of these groups at the end of the year were better than those previously presented from comparable studies (124, 259). All the patients had kept their motor, hand, and ADL functions reasonably intact, which must be said to be an excellent achievement.

Another weakness is the fact that the intensive exercise group did not comply one hundred per cent with the proposed interventions. This of course must be seen in the light of the fact that stroke is a complex disease with a heterogeneous population and development. In that respect we had a representative stroke population in our study.

One fact that might be considered a weakness was that some therapists administered a sub-maximal programme to patients whom they had volunteered to exercise maximally. This was explained by the therapists involved as being a practical adaptation to pathological conditions such as heart failure, pain and a poor cognitive status, which inhibited maximal effort. In order to carry out the exercises, adjustments were made so that routines could be maintained throughout the study period. This is probably also one of the reasons why so many patients complied with the exercise programmes.

7   Conclusions and clinical implications

* Physiotherapy treatment using the Motor Learning Programme approach is preferable to that based on the Bobath concept in the acute rehabilitation of patients with stroke.
* There is no carry-over effect of gains obtained during initial physiotherapy regimes on long-term function. During the first to fourth year after a stroke, with minimal or no intervention, there is a rapid deterioration of activities of daily living and motor function and an increased dependency on relatives. There is a gap between the acute phase with intensive treatment, and later stages with no or little follow-up of physiotherapy or rehabilitation activities.
* There is a strong relationship between the 6-Minute Walk Test and static and dynamic balance in the early rehabilitation of patients with stroke. This indicates that balance, both static and dynamic, needs to be addressed equally in the early rehabilitation of stroke patients, and is closely related to task, e.g. walking, getting up from a chair, turning, and reaching, and cannot be regarded as separate from the task.
* Motor function, activities of daily living functions and grip strength improved and were maintained during the first year after stroke in all patients irrespective of the exercise regime. This indicates the importance of motivation for regular exercise in the first year after stroke.
* A follow-up programme on a consultative basis is as beneficial as a compulsory exercise programme. However, the exercises need to be encouraged and instituted by medical staff with knowledge and an interest in intensive functional exercise programmes individually tailored for stroke patients.

8   Suggestions for further research

The results of this thesis indicate challenges for the physiotherapy practice and generate questions for further research:

First: There is a need, in both the acute and chronic stroke rehabilitation, for further development of effective physiotherapy programmes and task-oriented interventions that will enhance function, activity and participation, including quality of life, in patients with stroke. Preferably the development of physiotherapy programmes should incorporate questions on frequency, intensity, time and type of training in relation to patients with stroke.

Secondly: In order to develop these programmes there is also a need to further investigate instruments and tests whereby the progression of functions in patients with stroke can be evaluated and measured. Although several instruments are available, for example testing endurance, very few have been tried specifically on patients with stroke. There is a need to further explore how existing tests and instruments can be used in stroke care and to determine whether there is a need to develop new instruments to capture the specific problems in patients with stroke.

Thirdly: Although stroke research has developed immensely through the years, there are still very few studies describing the circumstances of patients with stroke and their relatives, and their new life with residual problems resulting from the stroke and the difficulties that might arise in all areas as a consequence of these problems. There is a need to investigate how practical programmes for stroke patients involving and carried out by their closest relatives, can influence the outcomes in all dimensions of health and coping, to sustain function, activity and participation.

In summary: it is hoped that this research will have increased the insight into the effect of different physiotherapy approaches and will have contributed to the development of evidence-based practice in physiotherapy in stroke. Aspects of motor function recovery in stroke patients in the longitudinal perspective have been described, and the results have hopefully contributed to the recognition of the importance of follow-up of patients with stroke. Furthermore, this work has contributed to the physiotherapy approach in the acute stroke setting, by elucidating the importance of task-oriented exercises and, in the chronic stage of regular follow-ups, which enhance motivation and coping strategies. This can serve as a model for physiotherapy rehabilitation of stroke.

It is hoped that the results of these investigations will be useful in the development of services, methods and outcome measures in care and in research in the future.

9   Reference List

1   Aho K, Harmsen P, Hatano S, Marquardsen J, Smirnov VE, Strasser T. Cerebrovascular disease in the community: Results of a WHO collaborative study. Bull World Health Organ 1980; 58:113-130.

2   The National Board of Health and welfare. Socialstyrelsen. Available from URL: http://www.socialstyrelsen.se/NR/rdonlyres/B9011B06-2FF8-4AA2-99C8-65C725C6CC76/4864/_20061021.pdf). Retrieved June 28/06/2006.

3   Ellekjaer H, Holmen J, Kruger O, Terent A. Identification of incident stroke in Norway - Hospital discharge data compared with a population-based stroke register 5. Stroke 1999; 30(1):56-60.

4   Astra Zeneca home site. Available from URL: http://www.astrazeneca.no/sykdommer/hjerneslag/for_helsepersonell/index.html. Retrieved 040706.

5   Wyller TB. Prevalence of stroke and stroke-related disability. Stroke 1998; 29(4):866.

6   Sarti C, Rastenyte D, Cepaitis Z, Tuomilehto J. International trends in mortality from stroke, 1968 to 1994. Stroke 2000; 31(7):1588-1601.

7   Immonen-Raiha P, Sarti C, Tuomilehto J, Torppa J, Lehtonen A, Sivenius J, Mononen A, Narva EV. Eleven-year trends of stroke in Turku, Finland. Neuroepidemiology 2003; 22(3):196-203.

8   Norwegian Institute for Public health. Available from URL: www.fhi.no. Retrieved 040706.

9   Stegmayr B, Asplund K. Improved survival after stroke but unchanged risk of incidence. Lakartidningen 2003; 100 (44): 3492-3498.

10   Stegmayr B, Asplund K, Wester PO. Trends in incidence, case-fatality rate, and severity of stroke in northern Sweden, 1985-1991. Stroke 1994; 25(9):1738-1745.

11   The national stroke register in Sweden. Riks stroke. Available from URL: http://www.riks-stroke.org/files/ENGcontents.html Retrieved 040706.

12   Stroke Unit Trialists' Collaboration. Organised inpatient (stroke unit) care for stroke. The Cochrane Database Syst Rev 2001, Issue 3. Art. No.: CD000197. DOI: 10.1002/14651858.CD000197.

13 Indredavik B, Bakke F, Slørdahl SA, Rokseth R, Håheim LL. Stroke unit treatment improves long-term quality of life: a randomised controlled trial. Stroke1998; 29 (5): 895-899.

14 Strand T, Asplund K, Eriksson S, Hægg E, Lithner F, Wester PO. A non-intensive stroke unit reduces functional disability and the need for long-term hospitalization. Stroke1985; 16 (1): 29-34.

15 SINTEF, Helse: Norsk Pasientregister. Available from URL: http://www.npr.no/som/som_rapporter.asp Retrieved 110806.

16 Kristensen DV. Å være sykepleier på akutt slagenhet: hva gjør sykepleie på akutt slagenhet meningsfull? Master´s thesis, University of Oslo, Norway; 2003.

17 St Olavs Hospital. Universitets sykehus i Trondheim. Available from URL: http://www.rit.no/StOlav/Aktuelt/Nyheter/Nyhetsarkiv/2006/nytt_norsk_hjerneslagregister.htm Retrieved 040706.

18 The National Board of Health and Welfare. Socialstyrelsen nationella riktlinjer før strokesjukvård 2005. Available from URL: http://www.socialstyrelsen.se/NR/rdonlyres/1C136023-A517-48B8-B4C2-FD220E5BA50/5386/rev_20061022.pdf Retrieved 040706.

19 National clinical guidelines for stroke. Royal college of physicians. Available from URL: http://www.rcplondon.ac.uk/pubs/books/stroke/stroke_guidelines_2ed.pdf Retrieved 040706.

20 Khadilkhar A, Philips K, Jean N, Lamothe C, Milne S, Sarnecka J. Ottawa panel evidence-based clinical practise guidelines for post-stroke rehabilitation. Top Stroke Rehabil 2006; 13(2): 1-269.

21 Field MJ, Lohr KN. Guidelines for clinical practice: from development to use. Washington DC: National Academy Press; 1992.

22 Bayona NA, Bitensky J, Foley N, Teasell R. Intrinsic factors influencing post stroke reorganization. Top Stroke Rehabil 2005; 12 (3): 27-36.

23 Bayona NA Bitensky J, Salter K, Teasell R. The role of task specific training in rehabilitation therapies. Top Stroke Rehabil 2005; 12 (3): 58-65.

24 Carr JH, Shepherd RB. Neurological rehabilitation. Optimizing motor performance. Oxford: Butterworth and Heinemann; 1998.

25 Lee RG, Vandonkelaar P. Mechanisms underlying functional recovery following stroke. Can J Neurol Sci 1995; 22(4):257-263.

26 Ward NS, Cohen LG. Mechanisms underlying recovery of motor function after stroke. Arch Neurol 2004; 61(12):1844-1848.

27 Trompetto C, Assini A, Buccolieri A, Marchese R, Abbruzzese G. Motor recovery following stroke: a transcranial magnetic stimulation study. Clin Neurophysiol 2000; 111(10):1860-1867.

28 Wiese H, Stude P, Sarge R, Nebel K, Diener HC, Keidel M. Reorganization of motor execution rather than preparation in poststroke hemiparesis. Stroke 2005; 36(7):1474-1479.

29 Hummel FC, Cohen LG. Drivers of brain plasticity. Curr Opin Neurol 2005; 18(6):667-674.

30 Dobrossy MD, Dunnett SB. Optimising plasticity: Environmental and training associated factors in transplant-mediated brain repair. Rev Neurosci 2005; 16(1):1-21.

31 Johansson BB. Brain plasticity and stroke rehabilitation - The Willis Lecture. Stroke 2000; 31(1):223-230.

32 Schaechter JD. Motor rehabilitation and brain plasticity after hemiparetic stroke. Prog Neurobiol 2004; 73(1):61-72.

33 Fisher BE, Sullivan KJ. Activity- dependent factors affecting poststroke functional outcomes. Top Stroke Rehabil 2001; 8 (3): 31-44.

34 Dishman RK, Berthoud HR, Booth FW, Cotman CW, Edgerton VR, Fleshner MR, et al. Neurobiology of exercise. Obesity (Silver Spring) 2006; 14 (3): 345-356.

35 Liepert J, Bauder H, Wolfgang HR, Miltner WH, Taub E, Weiller C. Treatment-induced cortical reorganization after stroke in humans. Stroke 2000; 31 (6): 1210-1216.

36 Lincoln NB, Gladman JRF, Berman P, Noad RF, Challen K. Functional recovery of community stroke patients. Disabil Rehabil 2000; 22(3):135-139.

37 Kwakkel G, Wagenaar RC, Kollen BJ, Lankhorst GJ. Predicting disability in stroke - A critical review of the literature. Age Ageing 1996; 25(6):479-489.

38 Wade DT, Hewer RL. Functional abilities after stroke - measurement, natural history and prognosis. J Neurol Neurosurg Psychiatry 1987; 50(2):177-182.

39 Schiemanck SK Predicting long-term independency in activities of daily living after middle cerebral artery stroke: does information from MRI have added predictive value compared with clinical information? Stroke 2006; 37 (4): 1050-1054.

40 Kollen B, van de Port I, Lindeman E, Twisk J, Kwakkel G. Predicting improvement in gait after stroke - A longitudinal prospective study. Stroke 2005; 36(12):2676-2680.

41 van de Port IGL, Kwakkel G, Schepers VPM, Lindeman E. Predicting mobility outcome one year after stroke: A prospective cohort study. J Rehabil Med 2006; 38(4):218-223.

42 Taub NA, Wolfe CDA, Richardson E, Burney PGJ. Predicting the disability of first-time stroke sufferers at 1 year - 12-month follow-up of a population-eased cohort in Southeast England. Stroke 1994; 25(2):352-357.

43 Wee JYM, Hopman WM. Stroke impairment predictors of discharge function, length of stay, and discharge destination in stroke rehabilitation. Am J Phys Med Rehabil 2005; 84(8):604-612.

44 Appelros P, Nydevik I, Seiger A, Terent A. Predictors of severe stroke - Influence of preexisting dementia and cardiac disorders. Stroke 2002; 33(10):2357-2362.

45 Nys GMS, van Zandvoort MJE, de Kort PLM, van der Worp HB, Jansen BP, Algra A et al. The prognostic value of domain-specific cognitive abilities in acute first-ever stroke. Neurology 2005; 64(5):821-827.

46 Hackett ML, Anderson CS. Frequency, management, and predictors of abnormal mood after stroke - The Auckland Regional Community Stroke (ARCOS) study, 2002 to 2003. Stroke 2006; 37(8):2123-2128.

47 Marsden JF, Playford ED, Day BL. The vestibular control of balance after stroke. J Neurol Neurosurg Psychiatry 2005; 76(5):670-678.

48 van Wijk I, Algra A, van de Port IG, Bevaart B, Lindeman E. Change in mobility activity in the second year after stroke in a rehabilitation population: Who is at risk for decline? Arch Phys Med Rehabil 2006; 87(1):45-50.

49 Heiss WD, Kessler J, Karbe H, Fink GR, Pawlik G. Cerebral glucose-metabolism as a predictor of recovery from aphasia in ischemic stroke. Arch Neurol 1993; 50(9):958-964.

50 Jongbloed L. Problems of methodological heterogeneity in studies predicting disability after stroke. Stroke 1990; 21(9):32-34.

51 Cramer SC. Changes in motor system function and recovery after stroke. Restor Neurol Neurosci 2004; 22(3-5):231-238.

52 Cramer SC. Functional imaging in stroke recovery. Stroke 2004; 35(11):2695-2698.

53 Petty GW, Brown RD, Whisnant JP, Sicks JD, O´Fallon WM, Wiebers DO. Ischemic stroke subtypes - A population-based study of functional outcome, survival, and recurrence. Stroke 2000; 31(5):1062-1068.

54 Jamrozik K, Broadhurst RJ, Lai N, Hankey GJ, Burvill PW, Anderson CS. Trends in the incidence, severity, and short-term outcome of stroke in Perth, Western Australia. Stroke 1999; 30(10):2105-2111.

55 Jorgensen HS, Nakayama H, Raaschou HO, Vive-Larsen J, Stoier M, Olsen TS. Outcome and time course of recovery in stroke. Part I: Outcome. The Copenhagen Stroke Study. Arch Phys Med Rehabil 1995; 76: 399 – 405.

56 Naess H, Waje-Andreassen U, Thommasen L, Nyland H, Myhr KM. Health-related quality of life among young adults with ischemic stroke on long-term follow-up. Stroke 2006; 37 (5):1232-1236.

57 Rosenvinge BH, Rosenvinge JH. Occurrence of depression in the elderly - a systematic review of 55 prevalence studies 1990-2001. Tidsskr Nor Laegeforen 2003; 3; 123 (7): 928-929.

58 Dam H. Depression in stroke patients 7 years following stroke. Acta Psychiatr Scand 2001; 103 (4): 287-293.

59 Appelros P, Karlsson GM, Seiger A, Nydevik I. Neglect and anosognosia after first-ever stroke: Incidence and relationship to disability. J Rehabil Med 2002; 34(5):215-220.

60 Langhorne P, Stott DJ, Robertson L, MacDonald J, Jones L, McAlpine C et al. Medical complications after stroke: a multicenter study. Stroke 2000; 31 (6): 1223-1229.

61 Zorowitz RD, Gross E, Polinski DM. The stroke survivor. Disabil Rehabil 2002; 24(13):666-679.

62 Kelly J, Rudd A, Lewis RR, Coshall C, Moody A, Hunt BJ. Venous thromboembolism after acute ischemic stroke - A prospective study using magnetic resonance direct thrombus imaging. Stroke 2004; 35(10):2320-2325.

63 Brott T. Prevention and management of medical complications of the hospitalized elderly stroke patient. Clin Geriatr Med 1991; 7 (3):475-482.

64 Lawrence ES, Coshall C, Dundas R, Stewart J, Rudd AG, Howard R et al. Estimates of the prevalence of acute stroke impairments and disability in a multiethnic population. Stroke 2001; 32(6):1279-1284.

65 Gamble GE, Barberan E, Bowsher D, Tyrrell PJ, Jones AKP. Post stroke shoulder pain: more common than previously realized. Euro J Pain 2000; 4(3):313-315.

66 Jonsson AC, Lindgren I, Hallstrom B, Norrving B, Lindgren A. Prevalence and intensity of pain after stroke: a population based study focusing on patients' perspectives. J Neurol Neurosurg Psychiatry 2006; 77(5):590-595.

67 Harari D, Coshall C, Rudd AG, Wolfe CDA. New-onset fecal incontinence after stroke - Prevalence, natural history, risk factors, and impact. Stroke 2003; 34(1):144-150.

68 Mann G. Review of reports on relative prevalence of swallowing disorders after acute stroke (Dysphagia 16:141-142, 2001). Dysphagia 2002; 17(1):81-82.

69 Sommerfeld DK, Eek EUB, Svensson AK, Holmqvist LW, von Arbin MH. Spasticity after stroke - Its occurrence and association with motor impairments and activity limitations. Stroke 2004; 35(1):134-139.

70 MacKay-Lyons MJ, Makrides L. Exercise capacity early after stroke. Arch Phys Med Rehabil 2002; 83(12):1697-1702.

71 Sezer N, Ordu NK, Sutbeyaz ST, Koseoglu BF. Cardiopulmonary and metabolic responses to maximum exercise and aerobic capacity in hemiplegic patients. Funct Neurol 2004; 19(4):233-238.

72 Canning CG, Ada L, O'Dwyer N. Slowness to develop force contributes to weakness after stroke. Arch Phys Med Rehabil 1999; 80(1):66-70.

73 Bohannon RW. Relative decreases in knee extension torque with increased knee extension velocities in stroke patients with hemiparesis. Phys Ther 1987; 67(8):1218-1220.

74 Tanaka S, Hachisuka K, Ogata H. Muscle strength of trunk flexion-extension in post-stroke hemiplegic patients. Am J Phys Med Rehabil1998; 77(4):288-290.

75 Newham DJ, Hsiao SF. Knee muscle isometric strength, voluntary activation and antagonist co-contraction in the first six months after stroke. Disabil Rehabil 2001; 23(9):379-386.

76 Fujitani J, Ishikawa T, Akai M, Kakurai S. Influence of daily activity on chances in physical fitness for people with post-stroke hemiplegia. Am J Phys Med Rehabil 1999; 78(6):540-544.

77 Winstein CJ, Rose DK, Tan SM, Lewthwaite RC, Chui HC, Azen SP. A randomized controlled comparison of upper-extremity rehabilitation strategies in acute stroke: A

pilot study of immediate and long-term outcomes. Arch Phys Med Rehabil 2004; 85(4):620-628.

78 World Health Organization, World Health Organization Constitution, Basic Documents. Geneva:WHO 1948. Available from URL: http://www.who.int/about/definition/en/print.html Retrieved 040706.

79 WHO ICF homepage. Available from URL: http://www3.who.int/icf/icftemplate.cfm Retrieved 280606.

80 Bonita R, Beaglehole R. Recovery of motor function after stroke. Stroke 1988; 19(12):1497-1500.

81 Ward NS, Cohen LG. Mechanisms underlying recovery of motor function after stroke. Arch Neurol 2004; 61(12):1844-1848.

82 Engardt M, Grimby G. Adapted exercise important after stroke. Acute and long-term effects of different training programs. Lakartidningen, 2005; 102 (6): 392-394.

83 Odwyer NJ, Ada L, Neilson PD. Spasticity and muscle contracture following stroke. Brain 1996; 119:1737-1749.

84 Carr JH, Shepherd RB. A Motor Relearning Programme. London: William Heinemann Medical Books; 1987.

85 Fellows SJ, Ross HF, Thilmann AF. The limitations of the tendon jerk as a marker of pathological stretch reflex activity in human spasticity. J Neurol Neurosurg Psychiatry 1993; 56(5):531-537.

86 Watkins CL, Leathley MJ, Gregson JM, Moore AP, Smith TL, Sharma AK. Prevalence of spasticity post stroke. Clin Rehabil 2002; 16(5):515-522.

87 Welmer AK, von Arbin M, Holmqvist LW, Sommerfeld DK. Spasticity and its association with functioning and health-related quality of life 18 months after stroke. Cerebrovasc Dis 2006; 21(4):247-253.

88 Thomas LH, Barrett J, Cross S, French B, Leathley M, Sutton C et al. Prevention and treatment of urinary incontinence after stroke in adults. Cochrane Database of Systematic Reviews 2005 ;(3) Art. No.: CD004462. DOI: 10.1002/14651858.CD004462.pub2.

89 Thomas LH, Barrett J, Cross S French B, Leathley M, Sutton C +et al. Prevention and treatment of urinary incontinence after stroke in adults. Stroke 2006; 37(3):929-930.

90 Jorgensen L, Engstad T, Jacobsen BK. Self-reported urinary incontinence in noninstitutionalized long-term stroke survivors: A population-based study. Archives of Phys Med Rehabil 2005; 86(3):416-420.

91 Harari D, Norton C, Lockwood L, Swift C. Treatment of constipation and fecal incontinence in stroke patients - Randomized controlled trial. Stroke 2004; 35(11):2549-2555.

92 Shumway-Cook A, Wollacott M. Motor control. Theory and practical applications. Baltimore, MD: Lippincott Williams & Wilkins; 2001. pp 274-280.

93 Horak FB, Shupert CL, Mirka A. Components of postural dyscontrol in the elderly - a review. Neurobiol Aging 1989; 10(6):727-738.

94 Bonan I, Derighetti F, Gellez-Leman M-C, Bradai N, Yelnik A. Dépendence visuelle après accident vasculaire cerebral recent. Ann Readapt Med Phys 2006; 49:166-171.

95 Marigold DS, Eng JJ. The relationship of asymmetric weight-bearing with postural sway and visual reliance in stroke. Gait Posture 2006; 23(2):249-255.

96 Zhang X, Kedar S, Lynn MJ, Newman NJ, Biousse V. Homonymous hemianopias - Clinical-anatomic correlations in 904 cases. Neurol 2006; 66(6):906-910.

97 Carey LM, Matyas TA, Oke LE. Sensory loss in stroke patients - effective training of tactile and proprioceptive discrimination. Arch Phys Med Rehabil 1993; 74(6):602-611.

98 Winward CE, Halligan PW, Wade DT. Current practice and clinical relevance of somatosensory assessment after stroke. Clin Rehabil 1999; 13(1):48-55.

99 Landau WM, Wetzel RD. Influence of somatosensory input on motor function in patients with chronic stroke. Ann Neurol 2005; 57(3):465-466.

100 Floel A, Nagorsen U, Werhahn KJ, Ravindran S, Birbaumer N, Knecht S et al. Influence of somatosensory input on motor function in patients with chronic stroke. Ann Neurol 2004; 56(2):206-212.

101 Hénon H. Pain after stroke: a neglected issue. J Neurol Neurosurg Psychiatry 2006; 77 (5): 569.

102 Turner-Stokes L, Jackson D. Shoulder pain after stroke: a review of the evidence base to inform the development of an integrated care pathway. Clin Rehabil 2002; 16(3):276-298.

103 Ada L, Foongchomcheay A, Canning C. Supportive devices for preventing and treating subluxation of the shoulder after stroke. Cochrane Database of Systematic Reviews 2005, Issue 1. Art. No.: CD003863. DOI: 10.1002/14651858.CD003863.pub2.

104 Baptista MV, van Melle G, Bogousslavsky J. Prediction of in-hospital mortality after first-ever stroke: the Lausanne Stroke Registry. J Neurol Sci 1999; 166(2):107-114.

105 Donkervoort M, Dekker J, van den Ende E, Stehmann-Saris JC, Deelman BG. Prevalence of apraxia among patients with a first left hemisphere stroke in rehabilitation centres and nursing homes. Clin Rehabil 2000; 14(2):130-136.

106 Fure B, Wyller TB, Engedal K, Thommessen B. Emotional symptoms in acute ischemic stroke. Int J Geriatr Psychiatry 2006; 21(4):382-387.

107 Meijer R, van Limbeek J, Peusens G, Rulkens M, Dankhoor K, Vermeulen M et al. The Stroke unit Discharge Guideline, a prognostic framework for the discharge outcome from the hospital stroke unit. A prospective cohort study. Clin Rehabil 2005; 19(7):770-778.

108 Morrison V, Pollard B, Johnston M, MacWalter R. Anxiety and depression 3 years following stroke: Demographic, clinical, and psychological predictors. J Psychosom Res 2005; 59(4):209-213.

109 Sellars C, Hughes T, Langhorne P. Speech and language therapy for dysarthria due to non-progressive brain damage. Cochrane Database of Systematic Reviews 2005, Issue 3. Art. No.: CD002088. DOI: 10.1002/14651858.CD002088.pub2.

110 Engelter ST, Gostynski M, Papa S, Frei M, Born C, Adjacic-Gross V et al. Epidemiology of aphasia attributable to first ischemic stroke: incidence, severity, fluency, aetiology and thrombolysis. Stroke 2006; 37(6):1379-1384.

111 Wertz RT. Aphasia in acute stroke: Incidence, determinants, and recovery. Ann Neurol 1996; 40(1):129-130.

112 Pedersen PM, Jorgensen HS, Kammersgaard LP, Nakayame H, Raaschou HO, Olsen TS. Manual and oral apraxia in acute stroke, frequency and influence on functional outcome - The Copenhagen Stroke Study. Am J Phys Med Rehabil 2001; 80(9):685-692.

113 Bell F. Principles of mechanics and biomechanics. Cheltenham: Stanley Thornes; 1998.

114 Pollock AS, Durward BR, Rowe PJ, Paul JP. What is balance? Clin Rehabil 2000; 14(4):402-406.

115 Marigold DS, Eng JJ, Tokuno CD, Donnelly CA. Contribution of muscle strength and integration of afferent input to postural instability in persons with stroke. Neurorehabil Neural Repair 2004; 18(4):222-229.

116 Geyh S, Cieza A, Schouten J, Dickson H, Frommelt P, Omar Z et al. ICF core sets for stroke. J Rehabil Med 2004; 36:135-141.

117 Geyh S, Kurt T, Brockow T, Cieza A, Ewert T, Omar Z et al. Identifying the concepts contained in outcome measures of clinical trials on stroke using the international classification of functioning, disability and health as a reference. J Rehabil Med 2004; 36:56-62.

118 Rasquin SM, Lodder J, Ponds RW, Winkens J, Jolles J, Verhey FR. Cognitive functioning after stroke: A one-year follow-up study. Dement Geriatr Cogn Disord 2004; 18(2):138-144.

119 Thomas SA, Lincoln NB. Factors relating to depression after stroke. Br J Clin Psychol 2006; 45:49-61.

120 Michael KM, Allen JK, Macko RF. Reduced ambulatory activity after stroke: The role of balance, gait, and cardiovascular fitness. Arch Phys Med Rehabil 2005; 86(8):1552-1556.

121 Lord SE, McPherson K, McNaughton HK, Rochester L, Weatherall M. Community ambulation after stroke: How important and obtainable is it and what measures appear predictive? Arch Phys Med Rehabil 2004; 85(2):234-239.

122 Mayo NE, Wood-Dauphinee S, Ahmed S, Gordon C, Higgins J, McEwen S et al. Disablement following stroke. Disabil Rehabil 1999; 21(5-6):258-268.

123 Jorgensen HS, Nakayama H, Raaschou HO, Olsen TS. Acute stroke: Prognosis and a prediction of the effect of medical treatment on outcome and health care utilization - The Copenhagen Stroke Study. Neurology 1997; 49(5):1335-1342.

124 Langhammer B, Stanghelle JK. Bobath or Motor Relearning Programme? A follow-up one and four years post stroke. Clin Rehabil 2003; 17(7):731-734.

125 Landi F, Onder G, Cesari M, Zamboni V, Russo A, Barillaro C et al. Functional decline in frail community-dwelling stroke patients. Eur J Neurol 2006; 13(1):17-23.

126 Jette AM, Haley SM, Kooyoomjian JT. Are the ICF activity and participation dimensions distinct? J Rehabil Med 2003; 35(3):145-149.

127 Perenboom RJM, Chorus AMJ. Measuring participation according to the International Classification of Functioning, Disability and Health (ICF). Disabil Rehabil 2003; 25(11-2):577-587.

128 Desrosiers J, Noreau L, Rochette A, Bourbonnais D, Bravo G, Bourget A. Predictors of long-term participation after stroke. Disabil Rehabil 2006; 28(4):221-229.

129 Schepers VP, Visser-Meily AM, Ketelaar M, Lindeman E. Prediction of social activity 1 year poststroke. Arch Phys Med Rehabil 2005; 86(7):1472-1476.

130 D'Alisa S, Baudo S, Mauro A, Miscio G. How does stroke restrict participation in long-term post-stroke survivors? Acta Neurol Scand 2005; 112(3):157-162.

131 Gottlieb A, Golander H, Bar-Tal Y, Gottlieb D. The influence of social support and perceived control on handicap and quality of life after stroke. Aging (Milano) 2001; 13(1):11-15.

132 Lindmark B, Hamrin E. Instrumental activities of daily living in two patient populations, three months and one year after stroke. Scand J Caring Sci 1989; 3 (4):161-168.

133 Sveen U, Thommessen B, Bautz-Holter E, Wyller TB, Laake K. Well-being and instrumental activities of daily living after stroke. Clin Rehabil 2004; 18(3):267-274.

134 Matsumori Y, Hong SM, Fan Y, Kayama T, Hsu CY, Weinstein PR et al. Enriched environment and spatial learning enhance hippocampal neurogenesis and salvages ischemic penumbra after focal cerebral ischemia. Neurobiol Dis 2006; 22(1):187-198.

135 Dobrossy MD, Dunnett SB. Optimising plasticity: Environmental and training associated factors in transplant-mediated brain repair. Rev Neurosci 2005; 16(1):1-21.

136 Rochette A, Desrosiers J, Noreau L. Association between personal and environmental factors and the occurrence of handicap situations following a stroke. Disabil Rehabil 2001; 23(13):559-569.

137 Teasell R, Bitensky J, Foley N, Bayona NA. Training and stimulation in post stroke recovery brain reorganization. Top Stroke Rehabil 2005; 12 (3): 37-45.

138 Shepherd K. Theory: criteria, importance and impact. In: Contemporary, management of motor control problems: proceedings of the step II conference. Alexandria, VA: APTA, 1991: 5-10.

139 Horak F. Assumptions underlying motor control for neurological rehabilitation. Contemporary management of motor control problems. Proceedings of the II steps conference, Alexandria, VA:APTA, 1992:11-28.

140 Woollacott MH, Shumway- Cook A. Changes in posture control across the life-span - A systems-approach. Phys Ther1990; 70(12):799-807.

141 Johansson BB. Rehabilitation after stroke. The plasticity of the brain is an unexplored resource. Lakartidningen 1993; 90 (30-31): 2600-2602.

142 Ernst E. A review of stroke rehabilitation and physiotherapy. Stroke 1990; 21(7):1081-1085.

143 Wagenaar RC, Meijer OG. Effects of stroke rehabilitation. A critical review of the literature. J Rehabil Sci 1991; 4:61-73.

144 Langhammer B, Stanghelle JK. Bobath or Motor Relearning Programme? A comparison of two different approaches of physiotherapy in stroke rehabilitation: a randomized controlled study. Clin Rehabil 2000; 14(4):361-369.

145 Stockmyer S. An interpretation of the approach of Rood to the treatment of neuromuscular dysfunction. Am J Med 1967; 46:950-955.

146 Voss D, Ionta M, Myers B. Proprioceptive neuromuscular facilitation: patterns and techniques. 3rd ed. New York: Harper & Row; 1985.

147 Brunnstrom S. Movement therapy in hemiplegia. New York: Harper & Row; 1985.

148 Bobath B. Adult Hemiplegia: Evaluation and treatment. London: William Heinemann Medical Books Ltd; 1990.

149 Plautz EJ, Milliken GW, Nudo RJ. Effects of repetitive motor training on movement representations in adult squirrel monkeys: Role of use versus learning. Neurobiol Learn Mem 2000; 74(1):27-55.

150 Kleim JA, Cooper NR, VandenBerg PA. Exercise induces angiogenesis but does not alter movement representations within rat motor cortex. Brain Res 2002; 934(1):1-6.

151 Jang SH, Kim YH, Cho SH, Lee JH, Park JW, Kwon YH. Cortical reorganization induced by task-oriented training in chronic hemiplegic stroke patients. Neuroreport 2003; 14(1):137-141.

152 Kleim JA, Hogg TM, VandenBerg PM, Cooper NR, Bruneau R, Remple M. Cortical synaptogenesis and motor map reorganization occur during late, but not early, phase of motor skill learning. J Neurosci 2004; 24(3):628-633.

153 Kleim JA, Jones TA, Schallert T. Motor enrichment and the induction of plasticity before or after brain injury. Neurochem Res 2003; 28(11):1757-1769

154 Petersen SE, van Mier H, Fiez JA, Raichle ME. The effects of practice on the functional anatomy of task performance. Proc Natl Acad Sci USA 1998; 95(3):853-860.

155 Ward NS, Brown MM, Thompson AJ, Frackowiak RSJ. Neural correlates of outcome after stroke: a cross-sectional fMRI study. Brain 2003; 126:1430-1448.

156 Classen J, Liepert J, Wise SP, Hallett M, Cohen LG. Rapid plasticity of human cortical movement representation induced by practice. J Neurophysiol 1998; 79(2):1117-1123.

157 Engardt M , Knutsson E, Jonsson M, Sternhag M. Dynamic muscle strength training in stroke patients: effects on knee extension torque, electromyographic activity, and motor function. Arch Phys Med Rehabil 1995; 76 (5): 419-425.

158 Pang MYC, Eng JJ, Dawson AS, Gylfadottir S. The use of aerobic exercise training in improving aerobic capacity in individuals with stroke: a meta-analysis. Clin Rehabil 2006; 20(2):97-111.

159 Kwakkel G, van Peppen R, Wagenaar RC, Wood-Dauphinee S, Richards C, Ashburn A et al. Effects of augmented exercise therapy time after stroke - A meta-analysis. Stroke 2004; 35(11):2529-2536.

160 Morris SL, Dodd KJ, Morris ME. Outcomes of progressive resistance strength training following stroke: a systematic review. Clin Rehabil 2004; 18(1):27-39.

161 Peurala SH, Tarkka IM, Pitkanen K, Sivenius J. The effectiveness of body weight-supported gait training and floor walking in patients with chronic stroke. Arch Phys Med Rehabil 2005; 86(8):1557-1564.

162 Macko RF, DeSouza CA, Tretter LD, Silver KH, Smith GV, Anderson PA et al. Treadmill aerobic exercise training reduces the energy expenditure and cardiovascular demands of hemiparetic gait in chronic stroke patients - A preliminary report. Stroke 1997; 28(2):326-330.

163 Forrester LW, Hanley DF, Macko RF. Effects of treadmill exercise on transcranial magnetic stimulation-induced excitability to quadriceps after stroke. Arch Phys Med Rehabil 2006; 87(2):229-234.

164 Macko RF, Ivey FM, Forrester LW, Hanley D, Sorkin JD, Katzel LI et al. Treadmill exercise rehabilitation improves ambulatory function and cardiovascular fitness in patients with chronic stroke - A randomized, controlled trial. Stroke 2005; 36(10):2206-2211.

165 Van Peppen RPS, Kwakkel G, Wood-Dauphinee S, Hendriks HJ, Van der Wees PJ, Dekker J. The impact of physiotherapy on functional outcomes after stroke: what's the evidence? Clin Rehabil 2004; 18(8):833-862.

166 Macko RF, Ivey FM, Forrester LW. Taskoriented aerobic exercise in chronic hemiparetic stroke: training protocols and treatment effects. Top Stroke Rehabil 2005:12 (1):45-57.

167 Pollock A, Baer G, Pomeroy V, Langhorne P. Physiotherapy treatment approaches for the recovery of postural control and lower limb function following stroke. The Cochrane Database of Systematic Reviews 2003, Issue 2. Art. No.: CD001920. DOI: 10.1002/14651858.CD001920.

168 Sackett DL, Rosenberg WMC. The need for evidence-based medicine. J R Soc Med 1995; 88(11):620-624.

169 Leung GM. Evidence-based practice revisited. Asia Pac J Public Health 2001; 13 (2):116-121.

170 Moseley AM, Stark A, Cameron ID, Pollock A. Treadmill training and body weight support for walking after stroke. Stroke 2003; 34(12):3006.

171 Zhang SH, Liu M, Asplund K, Li L. Acupuncture for acute stroke. Cochrane Database of Systematic Reviews 2005, Issue 2. Art. No.: CD003317. DOI: 10.1002/14651858.CD003317.pub2.

172 Martinsson L, Hardemark HG, Wahlgren NG. Amphetamines for improving stroke recovery - A systematic Cochrane review. Stroke 2003; 34(11):2766.

173 Bowen A, Lincoln NB, Dewey M. Cognitive rehabilitation for spatial neglect following stroke. Cochrane Database of Systematic Reviews 2002, Issue 2. Art. No.: CD003586. DOI: 10.1002/14651858.CD003586

174 Majid MJ, Lincoln NB, Weyman N. Cognitive rehabilitation for memory deficits following stroke. Cochrane Database of Systematic Reviews 2000, Issue 3. Art. No.: CD002293. DOI: 10.1002/14651858.CD002293.

175 Pomeroy VM, King L, Pollock A, Baily-Hallam A, Langhorne P. Electrostimulation for promoting recovery of movement or functional ability after stroke. Cochrane Database of Systematic Reviews 2006, Issue 2. Art. No.: CD003241. DOI: 10.1002/14651858.CD003241.pub2.

176 Outpatient Service Trialists. Therapy-based rehabilitation services for stroke patients at home. Cochrane Database of Systematic Reviews 2003, Issue 1. Art. No.: CD002925. DOI: 10.1002/14651858.CD002925.

177 Legg L, Langhorne P. Rehabilitation therapy services for stroke patients living at home: systematic review of randomised trials. Lancet 2004; 363(9406):352-356.

178 Vearrier LA, Langan J, Shumway-Cook A, Woollacott M. An intensive massed practice approach to retraining balance post-stroke. Gait Posture 2005; 22(2):154-163.

179 Mayo N. Rehabilitation outcomes in the 21st century: current successes & remaining challenges. ("what is in the spoon?") Final programme and abstract book. Stroke Rehab Gøteborg, Sweden; 2006: p 151.

180 Salter K, Jutai JW, Teasell R, Foley NC, Bitensky J. Issues for selection of outcome measures in stroke rehabilitation: ICF Body Functions. Disabil Rehabil 2005; 27(4):191-207.

181 Carr JH, Shepherd R, Nordholm L, Lynne D. Investigation of a new motor assessment scale for stroke patients. Phys Ther 1985; 65 (2):175-180.

182 Sødring KM, Bautz-Holter E, Ljunggren AE, Wyller TB. Description and validation of a test of motor function and activities in stroke patients. The Sødring Motor Evaluation of stroke patients. Scand J Rehabil Med 1995; 27 (4): 211-217.

183 Mahoney FI, Barthel DW. Functional evaluation: the Barthel Index. Md State Med J 1965; 14:61-65.

184 Hunt SM, McKenna SP, McEwen J, Backett EM, Williams J, Papp E. A quantitative approach to perceived health status: a validation study. J Epidemiol Community Health 1980; 34 (4): 281-286.

185 Berg K, Wooddauphinee S, Williams JI. The balance scale - Reliability assessment with elderly residents and patients with an acute stroke. Scand J Rehabil Med 1995; 27(1):27-36.

186 Butland RJA, Pang J, Gross ER, Woodcock AA, Geddes DM. Two-, six and twelwe minutes walking tests in respiratory disease. BMJ 1982; 284:1607-1608.

187 Podsiadlo D, Richardson S. The Timed Up and Go - A test of basic functional mobility for frail elderly persons. J Am Geriatr Soc 1991; 39:142-148.

188 Desrosiers J, Hebert R, Bravo G, Dutil E. Comparison of the Jamar dynamometer and the Martin vigorimeter for grip strength measurements in a healthy elderly population. Scand J Rehabil Med 1995; 27(3):137-143.

189 Poole JL, Whitney SL. Motor-Assessment Scale for stroke patients - concurrent validity and interrater reliability. Arch Phys Med Rehabil 1988; 69(3):195-197.

190 Halsaa KE, Sødring KM, Bjelland E, Finsrud K, Bautz-Holter E.Inter-rater reliability of the Sødring Motor Evaluation of Stroke patients (SMES). Scand J Rehabil Med 1999; 31 (4): 240-243.

191 Wyller TB, Sodring KM, Sveen U, Ljunggren AE, BautzHolter E. Predictive validity of the Sødring motor evaluation of stroke patients (SMES). Scand J Rehabil Med 1996; 28(4):211-216.

192 Wyller TB, Sveen U, Bautz-Holter E. The Barthel ADL Index one-year after stroke - comparison between relatives and occupational therapists scores. Age Ageing 1995; 24(5):398-401.

193 Finch E, Brooks D, Stratford, PW, Mayo NE. Physical Rehabilitation Outcome Measures. Baltimore: Lippincott Williams & Wilkins; 2002: Barthel Index: 87 – 90, Bergs Balance Scale: 93 – 94, Motor Assessment Scale: 169- 172, Nottingham Health Profile: 175 – 178.

194 Granger CV, Sherwood CC, Greer DS. Functional status in a comprehensive stroke care program. Arch Phys Med Rehabil 1977; 58: 555-561.

195 Larsen AI, Aarsland T, Kristiansen M, Haugland A, Dickstein K. Assessing the effect of exercise training in men with heart failure - Comparison of maximal, submaximal and endurance exercise protocols. Eur Heart J 2001; 22:684-692.

196 Leuppi JD, Zenhausern R, Schwarz F, Frey WO, Villiger B. Importance of training intensity for improving endurance capacity of patients with chronic obstructive pulmonary disease (COPD). Dtsch Med Wochenschr 1998; 123:174-178.

197 Kervio G, Carre F, Ville NS. Reliability and intensity of the six-minute walk test in healthy elderly subjects. Med Sci Sports Exerc 2003; 35(1):169-174.

198 Demers C, McKelvie RS, Negassa A, Yusuf S. Reliability, validity, and responsiveness of the six-minute walk test in patients with heart failure. Am Heart J 2001; 142(4):698-703.

199 Steffen TM, Hacker TA, Mollinger L. Age- and gender-related test performance in community-dwelling elderly people: Six-Minute Walk Test, Berg Balance Scale, Timed Up & Go Test, and gait speeds. Phys Ther 2002; 82:128-137.

200 Kelly JO, Kilbreath SL, Davis GM, Zeman B, Raymond J. Cardiorespiratory fitness and walking ability in subacute stroke patients. Arch Phys Med Rehabil 2003; 84(12):1780-1785.

201 Berg KO, Wooddauphinee SL, Williams JI. Measuring balance in the elderly - Validation of an instrument. Can J Public Health 1992; 83:S7-S11.

202 Tyson SF, DeSouza LH. Reliability and validity of functional balance tests post stroke. Clin Rehabil 2004; 18(8):916-923.

203 Mathias S, Nayak US, Isaacs B. Balance in the elderly patients: the "Get-up and Go" test. Arch Phys Med Rehabil 1986; 67:387-389.

204 Shumway-Cook A, Brauer S, Woollacott M. Predicting the probability for falls in community-dwelling older adults using the Timed Up & Go Test. Phys Ther 2000; 80(9):896-903.

205 Nordin E, Rosendahl E, Lundin-Olsson L. Timed "Up & Go" Test: Reliability in older people dependent in activities of daily living - Focus on cognitive state. Phys Ther 2006; 86(5):646-655.

206 Desrosiers J, Bravo G, Hebert R, Dutil E. Normative data for grip strength of elderly men and women. Am J Occup Ther1995; 49(7):637-644.

207 Merkies ISJ, Schmitz PIM, Samijn JPA, Van der Meche FGA, Toyka KV, Van Doorn PA. Assessing grip strength in healthy individuals and patients with immune-mediated polyneuropathies. Muscle Nerve 2000; 23(9):1393-1401.

208 Jones E, Hanly JG, Mooney R, Rand LL, Spurway PM, Eastwood BJ et al. Strength and Function in the normal and rheumatoid hand. J Rheumatol 1991; 8(9):1313-1318.

209 Hunt SM, McKenna SP, McEwen J, Williams J, Papp E. Nottingham Health Profile: subjective health status and medical consultations. Soc Sci Med 1981;15 (3): 221-229.

210 Hunt SM, McEwen J, McKenna SP. Social inequalities and perceived health. Eff Health Care1985; 2 (4):151-160.

211 Wiklund I. Long term follow-up of quality of life in patients with suspected acute myocardial infarction where the diagnosis was not confirmed. Scand J of Prim Health Care 1991; 9:47-52.

212 Ebrahim S, Barer D, Nouri F. Use of the Nottingham Health Profile with patients after a stroke. J Epidemiol Community Health 1986; 40 (2):166-169.

213 Gompertz P, Pound P, Ebrahim S. The reliability of stroke outcome measures. Clin Rehabil 1993; 7:290-293.

214 Visser MC, Koudstall PJ, Erdman RA, Deckers JW, Passchier J, van Gijn J, Grobbee DE. Measuring quality of life in patients with myocardial infarction or stroke: a feasibility study of four questionnaires in the Netherlands. J Epidemiol Community Health 1995; 49 (5): 513-517.

215 Brazier JE, Harper R, Jones NM, O´Cathain A, Thomas KJ, Usherwood T et al. Validating the Sf-36 Health Survey Questionnaire - New Outcome Measure for Primary Care. BMJ 1992; 305(6846):160-164.

216 Fillenbaum G. Multidimensional functional assessment of older adults. The Duke older Americans resources and services procedures. Hillsdale New Jersey: Lawrence Erlbaum Associates, Inc. Publishers; 1988: p 143-146.

217 Langhammer B, Stanghelle JK. The co-variation of tests commonly used in stroke rehabilitation. Phys Ther Res 2006; 11(4): 228-234.

218 Nagi SZ. Some conceptual issues in disability and rehabilitation. In: Sussman MD, ed. Socieology and rehabilitation. Am Sociological Assoc Washington DC 1965; 100-113.

219 Painter P, Stewart AL, Carey S. Physical functioning: Definitions, measurement, and expectations. Adv Ren Replace Ther 1999; 6. 2: 110-123.

220 Dorevitch MI, Cossar RM, Bailey FJ, Bisset T, Lewis SJ, Wise LA et al. The accuracy of self and informant ratings of physical functional-capacity in the elderly. J Clin Epidemiol 1992; 45(7):791-798.

221 Hoeymans N. Wouters ER. Feskens EJM, VandenBos GAM, Kromhout D. Reproducibility of performancebased and selfreported measures of functional status. J Gerontol A Biol Sci Med Sci 1997;52A:M106-110.

222 Gregson JM, Leathley MJ, Moore AP, Smith TL, Sharma AK, Watkins CL. Reliability of measurements of muscle tone and muscle power in stroke patients. Age Ageing 2000; 29:223-228.

223 Rantanen T, Volpato S, Ferrucci L,Heikkinen E, Fried LP, Guralnik JM. Handgrip strength and cause-specific and total mortality in older disabled women: Exploring the mechanism. J Am Geriatr Soc 2003; 51(5):636-641.

224 Snih SA, Markides KS, Ottenbacher KJ, Raji MA. Hand grip strength and incident ADL disability in elderly Mexican Americans over a seven-year period. Aging Clin Exp Res 2004; 16(6):481-486.

225 Kurillo G, Zupan A, Bajd T. Force tracking system for the assessment of grip force control in patients with neuromuscular diseases. Clin Biomech (Bristol Avon) 2004; 19(10):1014-1021.

226 Pandyan AD, Johnson GR, Price CIM, Curless RH, Barnes MP, Rodgers H. A review of the properties and limitations of the Ashworth and Modified Ashworth Scales as measures of spasticity. Clin Rehab 1999; 13:373-383.

227 Bakheit AMO, Maynard VA, Curnow J, Hudson N, Kodapala S. The relation between Ashworth scale scores and the excitability of the alpha motor neurones in patients with post-stroke muscle spasticity. J Neurol Neurosurg Psychiatry 2003; 74:646-648.

228 Tardieu G, Shentoub S, Delarue R. A la recherché d ´une technique de mesure de la spasticité. Rev Neurol 1954; 91:143-144.

229 Patrick E, Ada L. The Tardieu Scale differentiates contracture from spasticity whereas the Ashworth Scale is confounded by it. Clin Rehab 2006; 20:173-182.

230 van Vliet PM, Lincoln NB, Foxall A. Comparison of Bobath based and movement science based treatment for stroke: a randomised controlled trial. J Neurol Neurosurg Psychiatry 2005; 76(4):503-508.

231 International Bobath Instructors Association. Available at URL: http://www.ibita.org/ Retrieved 290806.

232 Liao YL, Mcgee DL, Cao G, Cooper RS. Quality of the last year of life of older adults: 1986 vs 1993. JAMA 2000; 283(4):512-518.

233 Kauhanen ML, Korpelainen JT, Hiltunen P, Nieminen P, Sotaniemi KA, Myllylæ VV. Domains and determinants of quality of life after stroke caused by brain infarction. Arch Phys Med Rehabil 2000; 81(12):1541-1546.

234 Van der Werf SP, van den Broek HLP, Anten HWM, Bleijenberg G. Experience of severe fatigue long after stroke and its relation to depressive symptoms and disease characteristics. Euro Neurol 2001; 45(1):28-33.

235 Nashner LM. Balance adjustments of humans perturbed while walking. J Neurophysiol 1980; 44(4):650-664.

236 Pedotti A. A study of motor coordination and neuromuscular activities in human locomotion. Biol Cybern 1977; 26(1) 53-62.

237 DeQuervain IAK, Simon SR, Leurgans S, Pease WS, McAllister D. Gait pattern in the early recovery period after stroke. J Bone Joint Surg Am 1996; 78A (10):1506-1514.

238 Cromwell RL, Newton RA. Relationship between balance and gait stability in healthy older adults. J Aging Phys Act 2004; 12(1):90-100.

239 Shkuratova N, Morris ME, Huxham F. Effects of age on balance control during walking. Arch Phys Med Rehabil 2004; 85(4):582-588.

240 Lamontagne A, Fung J. Faster is better - Implications for speed-intensive gait training after stroke. Stroke 2004; 35(11):2543-2548.

241 Eng JJ, Chu KS, Dawson AS, Kim CM, Hepburn KE. Functional walk tests in individuals with stroke - Relation to perceived exertion and myocardial exertion. Stroke 2002; 33(3):756-761.

242 Pohl PS, Perera S, Duncan PW, Maletsky R, Whitman R, Studenski S. Gains in distance walking in a 3-month follow-up post stroke: What changes? Neurorehabil Neural Repair 2004; 18(1):30-36.

243 Pohl PS, Duncan PW, Perera S, Liu W, Lai SM, Studenski S et al. Influence of stroke-related impairments on performance in 6-minute walk test. J Rehabil Res Dev 2002; 39:439-444.

244 Kandel ER, Schwartz JH, Jessell TM. Principles of neural science (4th Edition) Toronto: McGraw-Hill; 2000.

245 Cobb S. Social support as a moderater of life stress. Psychosom Med 1976; 38:300-314.

246 Johnston M, Morrison V, Macwalter R, Partridge C. Perceived control, coping and recovery from disability following stroke. Psychol Health 1999; 14(2):181-192.

247 Beckley MN. Community participation following cerebrovascular accident: Impact of the buffering model of social support. Am J Occup Ther 2006; 60(2):129-135.

248 Lawrence ES, Coshall C, Dundas R, Stewart J, Rudd AG, Howard R et al. Estimates of the prevalence of acute stroke impairments and disability in a multiethnic population. Stroke 2001; 32(6):1279-1284.

249 Dean CM, Richards CL, Malouin F. Task-related circuit training improves performance of locomotor tasks in chronic stroke: A randomized, controlled pilot trial. Arch Phys Med Rehabil 2000; 81:409-417.

250 Duncan PW, Horner RD, Reker DA, Samsa GP, Hoenig H, Hamilton B et al. Adherence to afteracute rehabilitation guidelines is associated with functional recovery in stroke. Stroke 2002; 33:167-177.

251 Green J, Forster A, Bogle S, Young J. Physiotherapy for patients with mobility problems more than 1 year after stroke: a randomised controlled trial. Lancet 2002; 359:199-203.

252 McClellan R, Ada L. A six-week, resource-efficient mobility program after discharge from rehabilitation improves standing in people affected by stroke: Placebo-controlled, randomised trial. Aust J Physiother 2004; 50:163-167.

253 Salbach NM, Mayo NE, Robichaud-Ekstrand S, Hanley JA, Richards CL, Wood-Dauphinee S. The effect of a task-oriented walking intervention on improving balance self-efficacy after stroke: A randomized, controlled trial. J Am Geriatr Soc 2005; 53:576-582.

254 Taub E, Lum PS, Hardin P, Mark VW, Uswatte G. AutoCITE - Automated delivery of CI therapy with reduced effort by therapists. Stroke 2005; 36:1301-1304.

255 Paolucci S, Antonucci G, Pratesi L, Traballesi M, Lubich S, Grasso MG. Functional outcome in stroke inpatient rehabilitation: Predicting no, low and high response patients. Cerebrovasc Dis 1998; 8:228-234.

256 Black-Schaffer RM, Winston C. Age and functional outcome after stroke. Top Stroke Rehabil 2004; 11:23-32.

257 Paolucci S, Antonucci G, Grasso MG, Bragoni M, Coiro P, De Angelis D et al. Functional outcome of ischemic and hemorrhagic stroke patients after inpatient rehabilitation a matched comparison. Stroke 2003; 34:2861-2865.

258 Ergeletzis D, Kevorkian RG, Rintala D. Rehabilitation of the older stroke patient - Functional outcome and comparison with younger patients. Am J Phys Med Rehabil 2002; 81:881-889.

259 Olney SJ, Nymark J, Brouwer B, Culham E, Day A, Heard J, Henderson M, Parvataneni K. A randomized controlled trial of supervised versus unsupervised exercise programs for ambulatory stroke survivors. Stroke 2006; 37: 476-481.

260 Altmann D. Practical statistics for medical research. London: Chapman Hall; 1991.

261 Pallant J. SPSS Survival manual. Second edition. London: Open University Press; 2005.

262 Tabachnick BG, Fidell LS. Using multivariate statistics. Fifth Edition. Boston: Pearson, Allyn and Bacon; 2007, 2001, 1996.

Attachments

Attachment 1

Physiotherapy Study I, Bobath or Motor Relearning Programme?

Both groups:

ADL activities:

Turn in bed
From lying to sitting
From sitting to standing
Standing position
Walking
Progression type even - uneven surface, variation of speed, walking stairs

Balance:

Do exercises in all positions according to programme / approach

Transfer:

Do exercises in all positions according to programme / approach

Arms:

Do stability and mobility exercises in all directions; frontal, horizontal and sagittal

Hands:

Exercises for gross and fine motor function

Trunks:

Exercises for stability and flexibility according to programme / approach

Legs:

Do stability and mobility exercises in all directions; frontal, horizontal and sagittal

Attachment 2

Physiotherapy group 1.

Motor Relearning Programme:

Dress during exercises:	functional and comfortable but the patient's choice
Time:	40 minutes
"Therapy style": coach	The physiotherapist takes initiative to and arranges the exercises, the patient is in command by expressing his / her goals, verbally and physically, according to what is most important to achieve for him / her.
Exercise premises:	Functional room; e.g. the patient's room, bath, kitchen; as realistic situation as possible

Exercises are characterized by:

1. "Hands -off" therapy wise. The exercises are arranged and supervised by the physiotherapist but the patient goes through with it.
2. Focus on the whole task and coping. How is secondary; increased spasticity and "pathological reflexes" is accepted as long as the patient can perform the task / function.
3. The therapist is not thinking of CNS as a hierarchy: if the patient wishes to try; we try!
4. Motor control theory according to the philosophy; stimuli acts on different systems in the brain and body; will power is the most powerful stimuli.
5. Assistive devices allowed according to the philosophy: 2any function is better than none".
6. Function / tasks are trained in ecological environment that is as realistic environment as possible in order to achieve maximal motivation and focus. The whole of the task is exercised / trained, not part of the task or function.

Attachment 3.

Physiotherapy group 2.

Bobath concept:

Dress: shorts or swimming suit, as undressed as possible in order for the
               physiotherapist to observe muscles and bodyweight position

Time: 40 minutes

"Therapy style"; the expert: The physiotherapist leads the exercises. The patient is the
                              recipient.

Exercise premises: The gym, therapy location

Exercises are characterized by:

1. Manual stimulation of the hemiplegic side type stroking, "clapping", use of weight
   shifting and shifting of the weight load. Stimuli according to the notion: right muscles
   should be manually touched; if dorsiflexion is weak, stimulation by hands-on to
   dorsiflexors!
2. Focus is always on the hemiplegic side; the physiotherapist always addresses the
   patient from this side.
3. The development of spasticity is closely watched by the physiotherapist. Pathological
   reflexes are inhibited, so called synergies, AR are not tolerated.
4. The development goes proximal to distal. That is; stability in trunk, shoulder and hips
   is of high priority. When this is achieved a more integrated movement is exercised
   type "wave with your fingers with straight elbow and flexed shoulder".
5. Therapy is based on a hierarchical development type children's motor development in
   the first year. Therapy is progressed thereafter; first turning in bed, sitting, crawling,
   and walking in that order…
6. Assistive devices are not allowed. The patient is not allowed to propel the wheel chair
   with the unaffected arm and leg see 2 and 3. If the patient needs support for feet it
   should be for both feet.
7. The patient is examined by the physiotherapist who evaluates the performance and
   develops the exercises in parts; e.g. hip stabilisation is trained in preparation for
   walking. When the patient is stable at the hip, the exercises are progressed till all "part
   training" is put together as a whole.

Attachment 4

Suggested components of the intervention programme

Time: 45 minutes

Endurance:

Intensity: HI - 70-80%, calculated from maximal pulse: 208 - 0.7 x age (Tanaka 2001) or 15 – 17 (hard to very hard) on Borgs rating scale of perceived exertion. At least two pulse peaks when training
ME – 50 -60 % calculated from maximal pulse: 208 - 0.7 x age (Tanaka 2001) or 12 – 14 (hard to very hard) on Borgs rating scale of perceived exertion. At least two pulse peaks when training

Proposal exercises:

- Walking
- Bicycling on stationary bike (arm- , leg- or combined)
- treadmill
- step
- working with balls or balloons

Strength:

Intensity 50-60% calculated from 1RM, dynamic, concentric and eccentric with preference for the last.

Proposal exercises: repetition 10 x 3

- **Extension of back:** pulley, pull-down, "walking stick", lying-extension.
- **Stomach**: ordinary sit-ups with fixation of pelvis if necessary
- **Arms**: push-ups in chair, weight –lifting, water bottles, pulley
- **Hips-legs**: ordinary knee flexion / extension, walking stairs, steps
- **Legs-feet**: toe-and heel rise on the floor, step, Airex mat, with or without support

Balance:

Maximal level on Borg: Varied with increasing difficulty: more or less visual input, visual or auditory "disturbances", obstacles.

Proposal exercises:

- walking even / uneven surface
- walking in 8, keeping borders
- walking on a line
- dual task
- obstacles
- dancing
- tai-chi

If not possible with any of the above:

- sitting: senior dance, balls, balloons

Use breathing techniques, take breaks; especially with heart and lung problems.
Do light stretching on big muscles after the end!